THE
DANGERS
OF
CELERY

THE TOXICITY & RISKS OF EXCESS
CELERY JUICE CONSUMPTION

ASA HERSHOFF ND

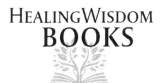

HEALINGWISDOM
BOOKS

Healing Wisdom Books / Asa Hershoff
321 N Pass Ave, Ste 151
Burbank, CA /91505
www.HealingWisdomBooks.com
www.asahershoff.com

Cover and Book Design ©2019 Asa Hershoff
Line Illustrations ©2019 Asa Hershoff

Ordering Information:

Quantity sales. Special discounts are available on quantity purchases by corporations, associations, and others. For details, contact the "Sales Department" at the address above.

The Dangers of Celery / Asa Hershoff —1st ed.
ISBN-13: 978-0-9841239-0-2

Table of Contents

Table of Contents .... *v*

Preface .... *v*

How to Use This Book .... *viii*

Part 1: A Medicine Called Celery *1*

Introduction...*2*

Food is Not Medicine..................................*5*

Celery Background Check........................ *13*

Celery's Nasty Cousins *18*

Health Claims *24*

Part 2: Celery's Dangers.................*31*

1. Allergy & Anaphylaxis...........................*32*

2. Light Toxicity...*38*

3. Suppressed Detoxification.................. *46*

4. Drug Interactions *50*

5. Nitrites *55*

6-8. Reproductive Health *60*

9. Low Blood Pressure.............................*63*

10. Bleeding Time *65*

11. Thyroid Disruption *67*

12. Kidney Inflammation *69*

13. Pesticide Residue 70

14. Heavy Metals...72

15. Homeopathy & Microtoxicity 75

16. Neurotoxicity...81

Part 3: Celery Truths & Myths 83

Nutritional Myths..84

Benefits & Caveats..94

Animal Studies 96

Anti-Microbial Action 99

Blood Pressure 100

Blood Sugar..100

Brain Conditions...101

Cancer..102

Cholesterol..105

Detoxification 105

Liver Function 106

Male Fertility 107

Stomach Acid 107

Part 4: Conclusion 109

Final Thoughts...110

About the Author...113

Index 114

Healing Wisdom Books 124

Preface

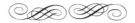

I have always had a deep affinity for plants, and a special relationship to the celery family—the Umbelliferae or Apiaceae. One of my great joys in the early days of my career was taking students on field trips to identify wild plants, both edible and medicinal. Among our finds were the ubiquitous wild carrot, wild fennel, and the look-alike killers of the family, poison hemlock and water hemlock. As my homeopathic practice progressed, I delved into the nature of plant families and the similarities in form, biochemistry and healing potential that lives within related species of foods, herbal medicines and toxic plants.

The celery family was amongst a small group that I studied intensively, including their botany and medicinal effects, but also their history, mythology and even spiritual meanings (anthroposophists Rudolf Steiner and Wilhelm Pelikan being a rich source). I lectured on the Umbelliferae to homeopathic students and went far towards completing a book solely on those airy plants. The pictures in this book are remnants of that unfinished work, drawn some 20 years ago. I am glad to revisit the Apiaceae in quite a different context, though hopefully with as much benefit as the original writings.

A Heritage of Natural Medicine

The title of this book sounds ominous. Nevertheless, it is a profound endorsement of functional medicine and natural healing and various holistic methods that are outside the scope of the pharmaceutical approach to health and illness. But it is also a cautionary tale. On the one hand, mainstream medicine has some basic problems, with its high tech diagnosis and low tech drug therapy. Its focus on treating the symptoms, rather than deeper levels of cause, is based on an incomplete understanding of health and how to promote healing within the body. And there is a serious failure to integrate the wide range of proven holistic treatments that avoid the risk of toxic side effects. On the other hand, commercialism, hype and overdone claims around diet or this or that supplement can put us into a fog of confusion and misleading information. In the end, this does not help the cause of natural medicine or a health-based lifestyle. It detracts from the real value of food and nutrition's essential role in the prevention and treatment of disease. And so a balance is needed. With holistic and complementary medicine, we have the possibility of taking from the best of both worlds. We can fully appreciate the biological sciences and solid scientific evidence, but also do a deep dive into the discoveries of biophysics, mindbody healing and cutting-edge nutrition.

Walking the Tightrope

Over the decades, some aspects of holistic and naturopathic health care have been adopted by mainstream medicine, with modern science validating what biological-based healing has been doing for hundreds (and in some cases thousands) of years. Some methods remain on the fringe. Yet with the emergence of genetic-based (genomic) nutrition, the age old practice of diet and nutrition is poised to become the most scientific form of medicine in existence, with the ability to precisely target our inherent biological weaknesses and tendencies.

Today we are also witness to an internet that has made a tremendous amount of information freely available on nutrition, herbs, homeopathy, mindbody medicine, meditation and energy healing—as well as disease treatment, prevention, and mainstream therapies. With all these competing voices, the ideal is a balance between science and tradition. This integrated approach can provide the optimal chance for individuals to make informed health choices and regain control over the future of their own well-being.

Asa

Asa Hershoff

Santa Cruz, 2019

How to Use This Book

This book contains four sections. If you are impatient to get to the specific dangers of celery, you can skip directly to Part 2, and then on to Part 3. Otherwise, you will find useful information and an important orientation in Part 1. Enjoy.

Part 1

The Medicine Called Celery sets the stage and puts forth the basic premise of this book: that celery is a botanical medicine that only recently was ported over to the food side of the equation. To that end we provide background on the Apiaceae family in general. There are also some thoughts on how to approach the questionable health claims that jump out at us from all sides. Bottom line, as a botanical medicine there is a risk-benefit ratio that comes into play when using celery.

Part 2

Celery's Dangers details the missing information on sixteen toxic risks of this member of the carrot plant family. For verification, and for those who wish to dig deeper, references to the related scientific research are provided after each of the topics. This is not a battle of beliefs, but a presentation of fact—and their proper interpretation. You can read straight through, or use the Table of Contents to jump to a any one of the specific chapters. This section also provides the additional, easily overlooked factor of microtoxicity: the evidence presented by homeopathic research into excess use of any edible substance.

Part 3

Celery Truths and Myths discusses some of the realistic science behind celery's possible value with references for further investigation. First the idea of celery as a source of vital nutrients is debunked. Then some of the commonly proclaimed benefits of celery are assessed, pointing towards some of the real value of this medicinal herb, but also why some claims are misleading or misinformed.

Part 4

The Conclusion summarizes our short but meaningful journey, to help put toxicity and benefits into both a scientific and traditional perspective. Apart from the hype or misleading contexts celery does have some place in a rational health regime or treatment protocol. There is a vast rainbow of healing herbs, spices, medicinal plants and botanical medicines. Everything belongs somewhere on that spectrum. The trick is to know where and in what proportion it is appropriate.

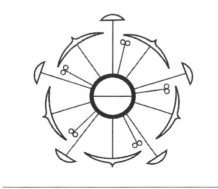

Flower Diagram of Apiaceae

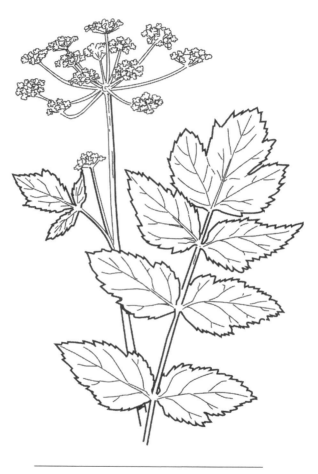

Pastinaca sativa - Wild Parsnip

Part 1

A MEDICINE CALLED CELERY

Introduction

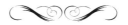

The Celery Issue

The point of this book is simple: To provide some important warnings and precautions regarding the excess use of celery and celery juice. Since time immemorial, there are plants that have been useful as medicines, and there are plants that are food. As one researcher rightly noted:

> Many people believe herbal medicine has no side effects and therefore they have a tendency to use herbs as an alternative medicine. However, using herbs may result in potentially dangerous side effects such as hepatotoxicity, nephrotoxicity, and altered thyroid function. (Maljaei, 2019)

Simply put, celery (Apium graveolens) is a medicine. It is a medicine that, due to careful selective plant breeding, is now used as a food. But like many botanical or herbal medicines, it has powerful biological effects. Using it in large doses, as if it were a harmless everyday food, is simply following bad advice. And as you will see, it is dangerous advice.

Information Overload

The explosion of health information in the form of self-help comes at a cost. Every year there are literally thousands of new books on the latest diet, nutrition or health innovations, both by knowledgeable individuals and by the copy-and-paste crowd. A simple Google search for blueberries, peanuts, vitamin C—or celery—can be frustrating. Trying to find out about a health related herb, supplement or natural therapy will yield everything from scientific evidence to outrageous claims, hype, fads, the latest in persuasion marketing, and the assurances of self proclaimed health-gurus.

There are useful websites and blogs out there, with health specialists offering straightforward advice for natural health consumers. But too often you will find this buried under an avalanche of several kinds of writings including:

- Breezy articles by journalists or health bloggers who are not professionals or experts in the field of health, but need to get out that next fascinating, topical piece.

- Information echoing other sites, with no personal investigation or in depth research—it's just news after all.

- Over the top enthusiasm, without either a traditional or scientific basis for claims or statements.

- Medical expertise that wears the robe of authority, but without any understanding or clinical experience of holistic principles (often the advisor for the above the journalists).

- Sites that have a strong bias towards a product or service, without concern for impartial information.

It becomes difficult and time-consuming to find a source of comprehensive or accurate information on natural methods of disease treatment and prevention. This is the reason why many earnest folks wind up with cupboards full of vitamins, supplements, powders and potions, unable to remember what they were for, or what value they bring to their journey towards optimal health.

Celery Drawbacks

That is the context in which we find ourselves. But in this book, we are focusing on hard facts about one single plant—celery. This would not be necessary except for its recent meteoric rise as a panacea, a cure for all that ails you. The current far-fetched claims of this herb could be ignored, except for the inherent dangers in this particular plant. No doubt there have already been many negative reactions in celery users since the craze began. But who would suspect this seemingly safe yet miraculous food? Who would attribute headache, insomnia, fetal abnormalities, seizures, miscarriage, life-threatening allergic reactions, heavy metal poisoning, accumulated liver toxins, or increased cancer risk to the simple celery plant? Armed with the knowledge contained herein, we can put celery into proper perspective. For some, it may also explain curious symptoms or unidentified illness that has cropped up since starting an intense celery juice regimen.

Apart from inaccurate claims, we will also look at the many myths that now surround celery, such as it being a rich source of nutrients, vitamins and minerals. As we will see, it is in the bottom tier of over 700 other vegetable products, some of which are 500 times more nutrient-rich. Understanding celery's minimal nutrient content as a foodstuff, and its side-effects as a botanical medicine, we can develop a clear view of its relative worth. It does have some real medicinal value, some of which we will discuss in this book. But in all cases the risk-benefit ratio has to be taken into account. Celery, as the cornerstone of a system of natural health, detoxification, or self-medication, is simply a mirage.

Food is Not Medicine

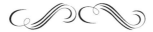

The Age of Misinformation

Fifty years ago, mainstream doctors scoffed at the idea that food had anything whatsoever to do with disease prevention, treatment or cure. Other than deficiency diseases, like rickets from vitamin D deficiency and pellagra from a lack of niacin, medical science knew less about nutrition than any 10-year old with an internet connection does in 2019. Tremendous progress has been made. Today the banner carried by the naturopathic profession for a hundred years has been taken up by functional medicine doctors. Medical colleges often include optional courses on holistic subjects. Even the term *alternative* medicine is being replaced by *complementary* medicine. The birth of the health coach—some well-educated, some just enthusiastic—has made personalized diet and nutritional knowledge more accessible. Health food stores exist in every mid-sized town and city. And you can log into Amazon and sift through thousands of nutritional or herbal supplements. If you want to go further, you can easily look up scholarly references and original research conducted in respected labs.

The "democratization" of health information out of the hands of a pharmaceutical-based medical profession, and into the marketplace, is a wonderful thing. But it has its down-side, as the amount of misinformation and disinformation is immense. One way to begin clarifying the confusing and contradictory landscape of facts and fallacies is to cur through this Gordian knot with a simple fact: Food and medicine are two different creatures.

Food is Not Medicine

It is logical to start with the oft-repeated quote, "Let your food be your medicine and your medicine be your food," attributed to Hippocrates, the so-called father of modern medicine. The only problem is, you will not find this statement anywhere in the sixty ancient texts comprising the Hippocratic Corpus. It was actually a health impresario who popularized the notion back in the 70's. As the researcher who investigated this misquote in detail stated:

> This literary creation is not only a misquotation but it also leads to an essential misconception: in the Hippocratic medicine, even if food was closely linked to health and disease, the concept of food was not confused with that of medicine.
> (Cardenas, 2013)

Still, it does make for a great slogan, indicating how important nutrition and diet are to our well being. Unfortunately it also promotes a modern fallacy. When we begin blurring the line between food and medicine, we run into trouble. This is not just a philosophical or theoretical issue, since the misunderstanding can have a drastic impact on the health of ourselves and our loved ones. In reality, food is not medicine. And medicine is not food. Having a healthful benefit does not transform a loaf of bread into a medicinal substance, except in a philosophical sense. There is not a single food that is not "medicinal" from that perspective, including water. But foods and medicines have different intended purposes, do different things in the body, and create different outcomes. In reality, plant-based foods and medicines exists along a spectrum. We have vegetables and fruits on the one hand, and botanical medicines on the other. While they do exist as a continuum, saying they are the same ignores the reality of botany and human physiology—and the purpose of language. If we extend this further, we can also put plant poisons at the far end of the same axis. And so it is crucial to know to which category a substance belongs, and where it fits in the overall spectrum. This sliding scale is shown in the diagrams below.

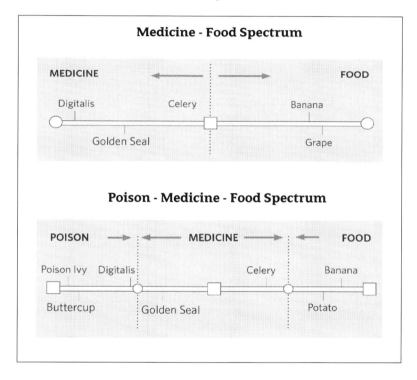

Though on the same spectrum, there is a big difference between food and medicine, even if both are plant-based. Foxglove (digitalis), henbane, the willow tree, the opium poppy and hundreds of other plants are the basis of important drugs still used in mainstream pharmaceutical medicine. But they also contain toxic components, such as poisonous alkaloids and glucosides, that can be lethal in the wrong dose. In some plants, one part is highly poisonous, and other part is medicinal. And in others, some of the plant is quite nutritious and safe, while other parts are flat out poisonous. The common apple is highly nutritious, one a day keeping the doctor away, so the saying goes. Yet a couple cupfuls of its seeds contain enough cyanide to kill a strong adult. At the same time, this is a cancer treatment of old, due to the cytotoxic properties of amygdalin in the seeds. Potatoes are fine, but don't try a potato leaf salad! Cashew nuts, with their peels still on, cause a severe poison ivy-like rash (since they are members of the same plant family). At the other end of the scale, some very dangerous, toxic plants have therapeutic value, while others are to be avoided in every circumstance. These divisions are part of the traditional lore of foodstuffs and the herbal medicine systems of China, India, Europe, the Americas, the Middle East and in literally every culture, time and place. But what then is the essential difference between food and medicine?

What is Food?

Food is defined as "any substance consumed to provide nutritional support, provide energy, maintain life, or stimulate growth." Hippocrates brilliantly described it as simply a substance that will be incorporated into the body's tissues, such as the nervous system, muscles and bones. To do this, it must contain adequate amounts of essential building blocks and nutrients, such as carbohydrates, fats, proteins, vitamins and minerals. While any food might be used specifically for healing, some are more potent in this regard. If you flip through Micheal Murray's *Encyclopedia of Healing Foods* (2014) or DK publishing's coffee table book, *Healing Foods* (2016), you will find nutritional and healing information on over 200 fruits, vegetables, grains, legumes, meats and more. The effects of these various substances includes everything from assisting weight loss, to hormonal balance, allergy relief, strengthening the liver, aiding memory and preventing heart attack or stroke. Of course these books are not comprehensive catalogs of all known foods, since literally every foodstuff used by humans has its own specific value. Still, of the 50,000 edible plants on the planet, only about 250 are under serious cultivation, and part of an established agricultural system. In comparison, the *PDR for Herbal Medicines* (Physicians Desk Reference) lists over 700 medicinal herbs in active use around the globe. Again, that is by no means a complete list.

We also have the new category of *superfoods*, which is basically a marketing concept, not a biological designation. The term indicates a substance that is either not part of our daily diet, comes from an exotic source, or has just been underrated till now. Still, this is an artificial category, as superfoods are either plain old food, or traditional medicinal plants. Another category that straddles food and medicine is covered by the meaningful and ancient term "spice." Spices are seeds, fruits, roots, or barks used as flavorings and food alteratives in various ways, often with antimicrobial or food preserving qualities. Culinary herbs like rosemary and thyme differ from spices only in the fact that we use a different part of the plant—leaf and stem —for their flavorful benefit. Curcumin (turmeric) is a good example of a so-called superfood that has a dramatic and very well-proven impact on our health. Both a traditional spice (curry) and thousands-year-old botanical medicine, it is not a food in the proper sense and won't be chopped into your salad anytime soon. Similarly, celery seed has held a place as a spice and medicinal herb throughout history. Being ported over to the dinner table is a recent event in its long journey.

What is Medicine?

To get a clear idea of the difference between food and medicine in general, we can look at the characteristics of plant-based or botanical medicines. We will see that they are distinct from food in their nature, and in how they are used, as listed below.

- Medicines do not enter into the composition of the body, like a vitamin, an amino acid, mineral or a fatty acid.

- They contain powerful chemical ingredients that have a drug-like effect i.e. glucosides, alkaloids, coumarins, etc. as major components of their biochemistry.

- Medicines have a much deeper and relatively swift impact on the body's functions, rapidly altering chemistry, physiology and even the structure of cells, tissues and organs.

- Technically, drugs are substances that activate or inhibit normal bodily processes and also bind to regulatory molecules in the body. In this sense, our own hormones and neurotransmitters are natural biological drugs or medicines.

- By their nature, all medicines have the potential for toxicity, or unwanted side effects, from mild to severe.

- All medicinal substances, herbal or otherwise, are dose dependent i.e. we should know exactly who is getting them and how much should be taken.

- Medicines are used for a specific purpose and a specific period of time—a treatment regime—or occasionally as a maintenance program, if necessary to maintain life and limb.

- Medicines have a wide variety of pharmacodynamic or biological impacts, which in herbal medicine are described according to their physiological effects i.e. diaphoretic (inducing sweat), antimicrobial, diuretic, astringent (drying), emetic (causing vomiting), etc.

On one end of the spectrum, we have botanical medicines with strong drug effects. They contain substances which have dramatic and deep action, and can be fatal when used in excess. Then we have milder botanicals with nutritive value that begin to approach the food category. At the other end of the scale, we have foods that are strictly nutritional, such as apples, grapes or broccoli. Some medicines have been hybridized over decades to push them more in the direction of food. Lettuce, for example, contains a milky sap that has significant opium-like sedative qualities and was even used as a substitute for scarce opium during Word War I. You will not find this *lactucarium* in the supermarket versions of romaine or iceberg lettuce, due to careful plant breeding. But let it "bolt" or seed on its own, and it will return to its former potency in a few generations. Note that this sap becomes biologically active only in the flowering stage of the plant.

Clearly, in the food-medicine-poison spectrum of plants, there are cross-overs and biochemical substances that share some categories. But the division is both physiological and practical. By looking at the Apiaceae (celery or carrot) plant family in general we can gain further clarity into the medicine-masquarading-as-a-food that we know as celery.

Research

Benzie, I. F. F. and Wachtel-Galor, S. ed.(2011). *Herbal Medicine: Biomolecular and Clinical Aspects. 2nd Ed.* Boca Raton, FL: Taylor & Francis.

Cardenas, D. (2013). Let not thy food be confused with thy medicine: The Hippocratic misquotation. *Journal of Clinical Nutrition and Metabolism (6).* doi.org/10.1016/j.clnme.2013.10.002

Glimn-Lacy, J. and Kaufman, P. B. (2006). *Botany illustrated: Intro-*

duction to plants, major groups, flowering plant families, 2nd Ed. New York, NY: Springer.

Gruenwald, J. et al (2004). *PDR for herbal medicines, 3rd.Ed.* Montvale, NJ: Thomson PDR.

Herman, L. (2015). *Herb & spice companion: The complete guide to over 100 herbs & spices.* New York, NY: Wellfleet Press.

Hock, B. (Ed.) (2005). *Plant toxicology, 4th Ed.* New York, NY: Marcel Dekker

Quattrocchi, U. (2012). *CRC world dictionary of medicinal and poisonous plants.* Boca Raton, FL: CRC Press.

Celery Background Check

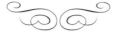

The Global Wanderer

To understand celery and its risks, it will help to take a brief excursion into the world of botany. We can touch on plant families, botanical medicine and even economic botany—how people have grown and distributed plants since the dawn of humankind. This is not for scholarly purposes, but as an important backdrop to understanding the safety of any food or herbal medicine, including celery. In our urban, technology-centered world, it is the rare few who have the time to forage for wild food or medicinal herbs, or have their own garden for that matter. A study of plants can brings us closer to our natural roots, and generate a deeper understanding of what we are eating and why.

It is useful to know, for example, that apples, pears, almonds, cherries, strawberries and a number of other luscious fruits, all come from the Rose Family (Rosaceae). And that this entire vast group of plants (some 5,000 species) produces no seriously poisonous plants—and just a few medicinal ones, *hawthorn* being the star. On the other hand, the common potato, chili pepper and tomato are part of the Nightshade Family with a large number of quite dangerous and deadly medicines. This includes the hallucinogenic terrors of *Jimson weed* and *henbane*, the seductive berries of *bittersweet* and *deadly nightshade*, and the very popular poison—tobacco. Even in the common potato, the relatively mild alkaloid toxin (solanine) is not destroyed by cooking, and will induce a subtle kind of aggression and dullness according to some.

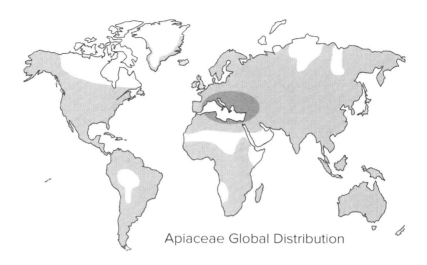

Apiaceae Global Distribution

In the Family

When it comes to the story of celery (*Apium graveolens*), we have a plant family containing many medicines and spices, as well as dangerous and deadly species. The *Apiaceae* or *Umbelliferae* group comprise some 3,700 plants, some which are well known spices, such as coriander and cumin, and others that have been tamed into vegetables, especially carrot and parsnips. Our central point is that celery itself is a medicine, and has been used that way since remote antiquity. Its role as a food is very recent, and it is clearly an experiment in progress.

Celery Mythology

With any food, its life in the wild and its history of use and cultivation can have unexpected twists and turns in its long journey to the dinner table. Originally from the northern and southern areas of the Mediterranean, celery is now grown everywhere, from North and South America to China, India, Africa and the whole of Europe. In that time it has accumulated its own lore and mythology, pointing in intriguing directions. Ancient Greeks associated celery with death and the underworld, decorating both graves and the heads of the deceased with it. Egyptians were using it similarly in their tombs over 4,000 years ago. Indeed, the saying "to need celery" meant you were close to death (not as a pick-me up!). Parsley was likewise dedicated to the queen of the underworld, Persephone. Because of these associations, celery was not considered an everyday food. Besides, its original bitter taste and fibrous stalks made it an unlikely addition to any meal.

Celery as Herbal Medicine

A few historical aspects of celery make its medicinal roots clear. Through the middle ages and beyond, *smallage* (wild celery) was used for a bizarre range of problems. It was once considered an aphrodisiac. Not to be outdone, a recent blog post touts it as the new Viagra. As we shall see, it is more likely to be effective for male birth control. Celery was also used to prevent hangover, for altitude sickness, and if that did not suffice, a few seeds in the shoe could help a person fly. There is a thread of meaning running through these claims, as they all relate to the simulating, traditional "Air Element" association of the Apiaceae plants. But like most traditional herbs, its actual medicinal benefit was often confounded by popular beliefs in magical powers and the reigning mythologies of the day. We know that in Europe the tomato (and potato) were banned by the church for several hundred years, and the plant that would be the red sauce known as ketchup was labeled the *devil's apple*—and considered lethal. On the other hand, potentially deadly herbs like henbane were used for toothache and to ward off the evil eye. This is one use that might be reinstated in the light of the heightened state of negative emotions prevailing in today's cultural climate.

Culpepper's famous herbal lists celery for detoxifying the liver and spleen, to be used even in the treatment of jaundice, for reducing gas, as a diuretic, and to help stones and gravel. Additionally it is named as a nerve tonic and blood purifier. It has also been used for the generic arthritic condition of rheumatism. Traditionally herbal medicines are described for their physiological effects, such as causing sweat (diaphoretic), fighting infection, bringing on a late menstrual phase (emmenagogue) or drying up secretions (astringent). But it is also important to understand that herbs are traditionally used in combinations, rather than singly, for a more comprehensive or synergistic effect. But whether alone or in combination, celery and all other botanical medicines are used at a specific dosage and concentration, and for a specific period of time.

Celery as Spice

Celery has been used around the world as a botanical medicine. As a food it was basically inedible. However, the whole plant family is highly aromatic, due to its internal essential oils. Thus its global popularity since ancient times lay in the seeds with their ample essential oils and flavonoids giving the characteristic taste and smell. Used as a strong flavoring it is a mild preservative with its antimicrobial and antifungal effects. The aromatic oils within the seeds of many species, including celery, coriander, fennel, cumin and dill, are a hallmark of the Apiaceae, aiding digestion and helping to keep food from going bad, especially during an era when refrigeration did not exist.

Transition to Food

As noted, wild celery was known as smallage from medieval times. The dark-leaved plant had long been used on the continent as an herbal medicine—first mentioned in 900 CE—but seems to have been put under cultivation for the first time in Italy in the 16th century. French and English gardeners began breeding the bitterness out of the plant, and it was being used as a salad dish in the late 17th and early 18th century. Yet it apparently still had to be blanched (boiling and discarding the water) right into the 19th century. By the early 1800's it was in America as well, and had its first big craze (but not the last) in the 1900's. History reveals that it was the third most popular snack in a New York bistro, next to coffee and tea, yet this novelty was more expensive than caviar. This is particularly interesting, since the whole effect of the aromatic plants in the family are as a stimulant to the senses, with a wake-up kind of taste and smell. Incidentally this again aligns with Steiner's view of the plant family as promoting the Air Element in the body, the traditional force of motility, creativity and action. Celery influences GABA, an important anti-anxiety neurotransmitter, but it also contains small amounts of potent neurotoxins known as polyacetylenes—stimulation indeed.

The root, celeriac, followed the same route in Europe, but has never been popular in the US or England. This is fortunate, since a common fungus that infects celeriac greatly increases its sunlight-sensitivity effect on people, a toxicity we will discuss further on. With the long process of selective growing and hybridization,the strong bitterness of the plant was reduced, and its sweetness increased. In spite of this, its medicinal properties—and because of that its inherent toxicity—remain intact.

Therapeutic Value

In modern times there are large amounts of research on the detailed biochemical effects of celery. The main concerns from a functional or holistic perspective are twofold. Does the substance just work symptomatically, or does it really cure an underlying imbalance or cause of illness? And does it have negative or toxic effects that challenge or even outweigh any potential benefit?

Either way, in spite of claims to the contrary, celery is no panacea. The search for the magic bullet that cures all illnesses has always been a dream of humankind. Like so many other plants, celery is a valuable herbal medicine when used appropriately. For example, recent studies show that it contains a compound which fights H. Pylori, the bacteria responsible for most cases of GERD (reflux) and stomach ulcers. Is celery the right treatment for these conditions? Another tree extract, *mastic gum,* is readily available in health food stores as a far more effective and well proven treatment for the same specific condition. And in this case the dosages and prescribing protocols are well understood, with no known toxicity. There is no single answer to all of humanity's ills and we will always have many therapeutic choices. For every condition that celery is purported to treat, there are sometimes hundreds of alternatives. And in some scenarios, celery's benefits are minimal or non-existent.

CELERY'S NASTY COUSINS

As we have mentioned, celery is a member of a unique group of plants, the Umbelliferae, so named because of the umbrella-like shape of their flower spays. But this isn't just any old plant family. Its 300-odd members includes carrots, parsnips, dill, parsley, parsnips, anise and fennel. Yet two of its species, hemlock and water hemlock, are in everyone's top ten list of the most poisonous plants on earth.

Conium maculatum (Poison Hemlock)

Hemlock is renowned as the lethal plant that ended the life of Socrates in ancient Greece. The method of capital punishment at the time was a mixture of hemlock and opium. The opium was merely a kindness, lessening the agony of death. With Conium itself, death can occur in a few hours from a paralysis that works its way up the body, finally shutting down the breathing apparatus. Native to Europe, it is now found all over North America. The *piperidine alkaloids* in the plant are equally lethal to human and animal species, pets included! When I and a colleague conducted herbal walks in the San Francisco area, many students noted that just brushing by the plant can result in feeling heavy and lethargic through the plant's toxic fumes. Apparently it can easily absorbed both through the skin and the lungs, so be careful. Celery also contains closely related alkaloids, that have various neurological effects.

Cicuta Virosa (Water Hemlock)

Related to Conium is the neurotoxic water hemlock. Also commonly found along streams and rivers, it is the most lethal plant in North America. As much as a few leaves will cause violent seizures and death through respiratory paralysis. Poisonings arise because the flower umbels look almost identical to wild carrot—except the latter always has one red flower in the center of the spray. This is a remarkable gift of nature that saves lives, if you know where to look. The cicutoxin in the plant is a polyacetylene, the chemical family in Apiaceae that has the ability to kill sensitive cells, including cancerous ones.

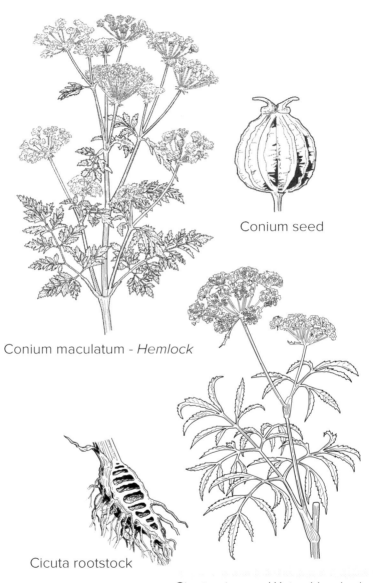

Conium seed

Conium maculatum - *Hemlock*

Cicuta rootstock

Cicuta virosa - *Water Hemlock*

Oenanthe crocata (Water Dropwort)

Water dropwort is considered the most poisonous plant in Britain. One of its white carrot-like roots or celery-like stems is enough to kill a cow, and accidental human fatalities do occur. In ancient times it was used in Sardinia, Italy, to execute criminals, and also to euthanize the elderly. It has also been used as an effective fish poison—for those without fishing rods.

Fool's Parsley (Aethusa cynapium)

Fool's parsley (aptly named) is sometimes called lesser hemlock, since it contains similar, but less powerful neurotoxins than hemlock. Still, accidental poisoning, as the name fool's parsley suggests, have resulted in deaths from mistakenly eating the leaves or roots. There are numerous other poisonous members of the family that we need not enumerate here.

Wild Carrot (Daucus carota)

The source of the modern cultivated orange carrot, this plant originated in Persia, but now grows wild all over North America and Europe. Apart from the easy confusion with its deadly cousins, it shares a few poisonous traits with celery. The leaves can causes phytophotosensitivity of the skin (damage from sunlight). And, with anti-fertility properties, it has been used as a traditional method of contraception and abortion since antiquity. The modern carrot, cultivated worldwide, was gradually hybridized over many centuries to create today's tasty root crop. The wild carrot is white and extremely tough, and inedible unless boiled sufficiently to soften its woody nature. Still, even here there are polyacetylene toxins which, though immunosuppressive and neurotoxic, are usually in too low a concentration to be harmful, but are disliked by cancer cells.

Parsley (Petroselinum crispum)

Parsley, like celery, will cause photosensitivity, and is especially toxic to dogs, being able to induce miscarriage, cause excess bleeding and resut in heavy metal poisoning. Animal research definitively shows that it is toxic to the liver and kidneys (hepatotoxic and nephrotoxic) and according to researchers "the plant should be kept away from pets and domestic animals." The light sensitivity effect is quite serious and can also permanently damage a dog's eyes. Oddly, there are articles all over the internet extolling the benefits of parsley for your pup. Commonly they confuse another even more toxic species with curly parsley, saying that the latter is safe. According to science, and the unfortunate experience of pet owners, this is simply not so. Other toxic members of the Apiaceae mentioned above, like hemlock, water hemlock, and water dropwort, are clearly dangerous for pets and have produced deaths just from digging around the plant.

While celery is not merely guilty by association, all these examples demonstrates that we are dealing with powerful medicinal and poisonous substances within this plant family.

References

Al-Achi, A. (2008). *An introduction to botanical medicines: history, science, uses, and dangers.* Westport, CT: Praeger Publishers.

Olatunbosun, B. S. (2013). Biochemical and haematological assessment of toxic effects of the leaf ethanol extract of Petroselinum crispum in rats. *BMC Complementary and Alternative Medicine, 13*(75). doi.org/10.1186/1472-6882-13-75

Peter, K. V. (2018). Celery (chapter 18) in *Handbook of Herbs and Spices, Vol 2.* pp 315-36. Cambridge, England: Woodhead Publishing. retrieved from: https://www.researchgate.net/publication/323691943_18_Celery.

Pizzarno, J., Murray, M. (Eds). (2013). *Textbook of Natural Medicine*, 4th Ed. St. Lois, MO. Churchill Livingstone.

Spiteri, M. (2011). *Herbal monographs including herbal medicinal products and food supplements*. Celery, page 33. Malta: Department of Pharmacy, University of Malta.

Witherall, R. *Spring parsley*. Retrieved from: http://www.pawsdogdaycare.com/toxic-and-non-toxic-plants/spring-parsley

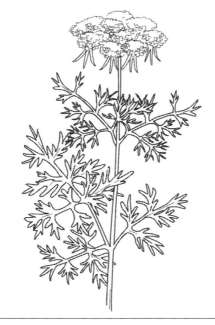

Aethusa cynapium - *Fool's Parsley*

Health Claims

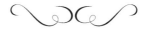

A Rock and a Hard Place

The average person, the engaged health consumer, is in a tough position. They need to be very savvy and well informed to navigate the mountainous landscape of advertising, marketing hype and flat out untruths that exists within the field of healthy eating, diet, supplements and self-care. How do we tell what is valuable and what is nonsense? Where is the balance between science and tradition, between the naysayers and those making outrageous claims? Sometimes it is difficult to discern the truth but fortunately much of the following advice is just common sense. However, in the case of health and healing information, there are still some special guidelines we can bring to bear.

Lack of References

Whether its a blog, an article, or an opinion piece in a magazine, if it does not contain any citations, no bibliography, not a single reference to where this information is coming from, it is simply not reliable. The same applies to any book on nutrition, diet or health recommendations. That doesn't mean that traditional knowledge, accumulated over centuries or even millennia, is not useful or valid. Personal experience counts too, as far as it goes. And knowledgeable experts may not have had time to quote their source. Yet it is the responsibility of the author or writer to perform their due diligence and fact-check before they offer seeminly definitive statement.

As we are all aware, fake news is the new normal and the rapid-fire news cycle means there is no longer the time or energy for media outlets to investigate. The science of social engineering began at the same time as the "age of advertising," when corporations and manufacturers realized that the public could be manipulated and influenced through emotional triggers and deeply ingrained fears and insecurities. Edward Bernays, the nephew of Freud, was one of the architects of this approach, and would be very proud of the modern world he helped create. Today a majority of blog writers, journalists and professional writers simply copy information from somewhere else. In this twitter world, there is little motivation to check sources or dig for facts. Mentioning a research paper or book is not a guarantee, but it brings credibility up a notch.

Exaggeration

Watch for superlatives. A food or herb can have "powerful" effects, be fantastic, amazing or awesome. But this has little meaning in sorting out the wheat from the chaff. Most importantly, beware of absurd claims. Consider the following:

> If you or someone you love has acne, eczema, migraines, fatigue, brain fog, anxiety, depression, bipolar, psoriasis, addictions, memory issues, Lyme disease, multiple sclerosis, cancer, bloating, SIBO, constipation, high cholesterol, diarrhea, heart palpitations, eye problems, or any other symptom or illness, celery juice is a powerful, foundational tool to begin moving you towards healing and symptom relief.

This is a direct quote extolling the virtues of celery juice. No one with basic health knowledge, whether a health care practitioner, holistic coach, product formulator, whole food worker, nutritionist, or health journalist would make such outrageous claims about any single substance, ingredient, or method. It is not only unethical, it is dangerous. And how about this one: "The Most Powerful Medicine of Our Time Healing Millions!"

Such statements do not have the authority of science, statistics, everyday fact, philosophy, religion or common sense. What they do is promote faddishness and gullibility, something we already have enough of in this world. If it sounds too good to be true...

Single Ingredient Conflation

On a more technical, but just as important point, describing the effects of a single vitamin, flavonoid, or mineral that is contained in a plant like celery, is misleading. Thousands of plants are screened by researchers for specific ingredients or biochemical substances that have some biological impact. Generally the purpose of this is to isolate the bioactive chemical, synthesize it, and create future drugs. Celery has a number of such medicinal ingredients, including flavonoids, glucosides, alkaloids and so on. But there are problems with then claiming that raw celery will do the same thing as a specific isolated extract, such as *luteolin*. For medicines like celery, that have a significant toxic component, it is not possible to get adequate amounts of trace flavonoids or terpenes without also overdosing on the negative aspect. Many of the experiments that show various physiological effects are done by injecting a single ingredient or a concentrate directly into a laboratory rat. While this is a good method to demonstrate toxicity or biological action, it does not emulate a curative effect through human consumption of raw celery. And as we shall see, celery is distinctly low in luteolin in any case.

Single Effects

The easiest way to tell a little white lie is to say everything nice about something, but carefully omit the negative. Most of us do this every day in a harmless way, whether about an idea, the clothes a co-worker is wearing or, if really polite, how I might feel today. Saying, for example, that celery can kill cancer cell is true, but that is because it is toxic and disrupts DNA and RNA. It is a killer. This does have an effect on viruses, bacteria, fungi, cancer cells—and human cells. There are many thousands of substances that can similarly destroy cancer cells, including the virulent drugs used in mainstream cancer treatment. Various lines of cancer cells, being of a primitive type, are more susceptible to such toxins. Deadly arsenic is one of the most ancient treatments for cancer, still used today to treat leuke-certain leukemias. Killing bad cells is a good idea, but by itself is far from a holistic cure, as the actual causes remain.

Single Therapies

There are hundreds of factors involved with health conditions. And every person is different and unique. Age, constitution, genetics, toxicity, past traumas, mindset, environment, all play their important roles. One size simply does not fit all. A coordinated approach to our health involves nutrition, diet, herbal medicine, homeopathy (essential in my experience) and symptomatic drugs if necessary. It requires physical activity, be it yoga, qi gong or aerobics. Mental hygiene, in the form of meditation, mindfulness or other kinds of inner work is crucial. In reality there are thousands of options that can be integrated for our unique constitution, proclivities, likes, hopes and dreams. Any claim that a single treatment or therapy is "it" is questionable, unless the "it" was had many moving parts.

Single (Wrong) Information Source

One of the truly humorous myths flying around various websites is that celery contains a unique pheromone, *androstenone*.
This makes it an aphrodisiac, as well as attracting the female
species. The fact that the role of pheromones is as yet poorly
understood, or that the stinky *underarm sweat* smell of androstenone is proven to be unattractive to women, is not the point.
The point is that every source making a statement about androstenone exposes the fact that they get all their information
by copying Wikipedia pages, not by reading original research
or through journalistic investigation. The androstenone Wikipedia page mentions truffles, pig's saliva, and male sweat,
along with "celery cytoplasm" as a source of the substance,
based on a certain (uncited) study. But a little digging (no truf-
fle pun intended) shows that in two major studies androstenone was present in *80% of all 128 plant species tested* (Simons &
Grinwich, 1989). Also, note that Wikipedia is user created. The
validity or veracity of the information is just as variable as the
person who posted it. Do you want to trust your health to an
anonymous authority? Or how about the ones who copy it.

Black and White Answers

Human beings are highly complex, and our organisms are incredibly so. Exaggerated statements that are highly polarizing
are either biased or misleading. Similarly, even with original
well-done research, the conclusions are rarely simplistic and
answers are often complex and multifaceted. Websites and
books often have a strong cognitive bias in selecting only the
answers they want. In the same vein, any promise of a quick fix
ignores all the factors involved in each unique person, and
casts doubt on the integrity of the fix itself. Generally, all forms

of advertising sell the same thing: hope. Unfortunately, playing on our weaknesses and fears is often effective but it merely continues to disempower our possibilities, and limit our ability to find meaningful, individual and unique solutions.

Authority Source

Authority is a huge topic in today's world of marketing, entrepreneurism, branding and so forth. Thus knowing who to trust and what sources are authentic has never been so important, or so difficult. First, we have tradition and the lineage of natural medicine. Men and women of great integrity have invested their lifetime in developing real expertise and even mastery of the subject, and those voices are to be sought out. At the other end of the spectrum is a sea of commercialization and marketing claims. But also there are earnest and even well-meaning individuals who have simply not paid their dues or put in the time to become knowledgeable.

Incomplete or misleading information is regularly put forth by pharmaceutical companies, but claims about natural supplements are not exempt from that possibility. In working with a dozen natural product companies over the years, I have found the majority are run by people with high integrity that believe in their products, often with a passionate commitment. But in the end it is "buyer beware."

Social Conformity

Lastly, and sadly, there is nothing more powerful than "social proof," the desire to conform, and the belief that, "if everybody is doing it, it must be good!" Whether you believe this tendency is fundamental to biological human nature, or a departure from personal intelligence, it is rarely a good thing. Following the crowd to the next product, fad or cult without pausing for rational reflection is not a strategy for success. Personal testimonials and stories provide inspiration, but leave us without any factual evidence. Endorsements of celebrities or highly satisfied customers are also a flimsy kind of proof. In the end, popularity has never been a litmus test for actual value or benefit. The ever-likeable tobacco plant still kills 8 million people a year worldwide, and dictators of the past have killed hundreds of millions. And they were very, very popular.

All these forces that seek to manipulate our minds and bodies can be cut through by our wonderful ability for careful and rational reflection and unbiased inquiry.

References

Cialdini, R. B. (2006). *Influence: The psychology of persuasion.* New York, NY: Harper-Collins.

Fitzgerald, M. (2015). *Diet cults: The surprising fallacy at the core of nutrition fads and a guide to healthy eating for the rest of us.* New York, NY: Pegasus Books.

Friedman, D. D. (2018). *Food sanity: How to eat in a world of fads and fiction.* New York, NY: Basic Health Publications.

Greenspan, S. (2009). *Annals of gullibility: Why we get duped and how to avoid it.* Westport, CT: Praeger.

Simons, R. G. and Grinwich, D. L. (1989). Immunoreactive detection of four mammalian steroids in plants. *Canadian Journal of Botany, 67,* 288-296. doi.org/10.1139/b89-042

Part 2

CELERY'S DANGERS

1

Allergy & Anaphylaxis

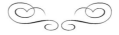

The Facts

The first and most pressing thing to know about celery is that it is one of world's most allergenic plants. Overall, food allergy is greatly on the rise, with an almost 400% increase from 2007 to 2016. In Europe celery is one of fourteen major food allergens that must be stated in the ingredient list of packaged foods. Indeed it is considered a serious problem in Germany, Switzerland and France, where one third of all anaphylactic reactions are due to celery. And here in the US it is considered that fully 30-40% of all food allergy reactions occur from celery.

Discussion

Allergy reactions are of four types, varying from mild to life-threatening. Type 1 or immediate allergy, involving igE antibodies, is the one we are all familiar with, from peanut reactions to hayfever. Celery sensitivity is more often associated with people who have existing pollen allergies and there is a crossover to birch tree pollen allergy, mugwort, Timothy grass, carrots and—surprisingly—apples. While one's sensitivity may vary initially, repeated exposure makes the reaction progressively worse. Pre-existing asthma or hayfever is also a strong indicator or risk factor that you may be predisposed to this form of food allergy.

Sensitivity happens from both handling and ingesting different parts of the celery plant, including the roots and seeds. Initial reactions may be mild, with typical symptoms such as tingling, itching or the onset of a skin rash. These are important indicators to avoid celery in the future.

If the allergic reaction accelerates, watch for these signs:

- Swelling, itching or tingling of face, lips, mouth or throat.
- Throat constriction and difficulty swallowing.
- Hives (urticaria or nettle rash) or local swelling of the skin, in any area of the body, after contact or ingestion.
- Asthmatic reactions, from mild to severe.
- Difficult breathing, from asthma or swelling of the throat.
- Abdominal pain with nausea or vomiting.
- Anaphylaxis or anaphylactic shock, a potentially fatal collapse of vascular and other body systems.

Allergy Defense

If you are diagnosed with a celery allergy or have had even a mild reaction, it is critical to be vigilant since celery extract or powder finds its way into numerous food products, restaurant meals, etc. Caution dictates having antihistamines on hand, though homeopathics are an effective line of defense as well. To deal with extreme reactions, allergic individuals should carry an EpiPen, an injectable which contains a mild dose of epinephrine. A shot in the thigh may halt a potentially fatal reaction. But if severe symptoms do occur, an immediate trip to the hospital is advisable and may be life-saving. Note that other relatives of celery are also high on the allergen list, including parsley. Some people are also deathly allergic to carrots.

Diagnosing Celery Sensitivity

How common is celery allergy? Statistics are hard to come by, but about five cases of deadly anaphylaxis from celery are known to occur annually in France, which has a fifth of the population of the USA. In some people this reaction only happens after exercise, so this is also something to watch for. Some individuals may discover the presence of allergies directly after eating. But, as is well known, allergy is often hidden and difficult to diagnose, while contributing to chronic health problems. A celery allergy can be diagnosed via skin tests (type 1 or immediate igE-based), or the appropriate blood tests to measure long-term IgG1 and IgG2 antigens. These last tests do not measure a true allergy, but certainly detect long-term sensitivities. If present, any level of allergy can have a significant impact on the immune system.

No one should begin juicing celery if they have a known allergy to other members of the Apiaceae, including parsley, parsnips or carrots. Even if you have never had an allergic reaction to celery, you may become sensitized by taking large doses for a prolonged period..

Celery Sources

Fresh celery is an obvious trigger for the allergy process. But while the raw vegetable is a common culprit, cooking does not seem to lessen the possibility of a reaction. The allergic factors are present in the highest concentration in the seeds, but also very much in the mature leaves and roots (celeriac) and lesser again in the stalks. Celery oil also has an effect, varying with the concentration of the active ingredients. This is problematic since it is the seeds that are commonly used to make the typical powder or extract that is added to many forms of processed or packaged foods. Celery in the spice rack is naturally from these aromatic seeds, as they contain the flavorful oils. Items that may contain celery extracts or powder include:

- Canned soups.
- Vegetable juice combinations (bottles, boxes, etc.).
- Bottled or canned sauces, including tomato sauce.
- Spice mixes or combined seasonings.
- Mixers for vodka, cocktails or other alcoholic drinks.
- Vegetable stock or boullion cubes.
- Salad mixes (packaged, restaurant mixtures, etc.).
- Stews, soups (processed, ready-made or in restaurants).
- Pre-prepared sandwiches.
- Vegetable chips or sticks (with rice, flour, corn, etc.).
- Marmite (yeast extract).
- Batter mix used in various frozen foods.
- Salts and salt substitutes that use a variety of vegetable powders, including celery.
- Essential oil of celery is also used in the perfume industry, though this will rarely be shown on labels.

Unfortunately, celery powder (and sometimes juice) is now present in a new form, providing a further hidden risk. You will find it being used in organic hot dogs and lunch meats, sold as "nitrate-free" products. This is inaccurate and misleading as discussed in detail further on. In this case we have both the allergenic factor and the potential toxicity of nitrates. It behooves the consumer to read labels carefully!

References

Anaphylaxis Campaign. (July, 2015). *Oral allergy syndrome.* Retrieved from: https://www.anaphylaxis.org.uk/wp-content/uploads/2019/07/Celery-2018.pdf

Ballmer-Weber B. K., Vieths, S., Lüttkopf, D., Heuschmann P., & Wüthrich, B. (2000). Celery allergy confirmed by double-blind, placebo-controlled food challenge: a clinical study in 32 subjects with a history of adverse reactions to celery root. *Journal of Allergy and Clinical Immunology, 106*(2), 373-8. doi: 10.1067/mai.2000.107196

Cianferoni, A. and Muraro, A. (2012). Food-induced anaphylaxis. *Immunology and Allergy Clinics of North America, 32*(1) 165–195. doi: 10.1016/j.iac.2011.10.002

Daems, D., Peeters, B., Delport, F., Remans, T., Lammertyn, J. and Spasic, D. (2017). Identification and quantification of celery allergens using fiber optic surface plasmon resonance pcr. *Basel, 17*(8), 1754. doi: 10.3390/s17081754

Fleming, D. (1990). Dermatitis in grocery workers associated with high natural concentrations of furanocoumarins in celery. *Allergy Proceedings, 11*(3) page 125-7. doi: 10.7326/0003-4819-105-3-351

Gawlik, R. et al. (2019). Asthma and exercise-induced respiratory disorders in athletes. The position paper of the Polish Society of Allergology and Polish Society of Sports Medicine. *Postepy dermatologii i alergologii, 36*(1), 1–10. doi:10.5114/ada.2019.82820

Gelburd, R. (Aug 21, 2017). Food allergies: new data on a growing health issue. *Food Allergy Research & Education.* Retrieved from   https://www.realclearhealth.com/articles/2017/08/21/

food_allergies_new_data_on_a_growing_health_issue_110709.html

Pauli, G., Bessot, J. C., Braun, P. A., Dietemann-Molard, A., Kopferschmitt-Kubler, M. C. and Thierry, R. (1988). Celery allergy: clinical and biological study of 20 cases. *Annals of Allergy*. *60*(3), 243-6.

Wüthrich, B. and Dietschi, R. (1985). The celery-carrot-mugwort-condiment syndrome: skin test and RAST results. *SwissMedicalWeekly,115*(11),258-64.doi:10.1055/s-2008-1069310

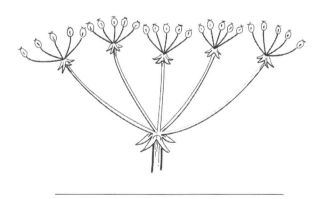

Umbelliferae Flower Spray

2

Light Toxicity

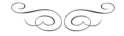

The Facts

Celery is one of a small group of plants that can cause extreme phytophotosensitivity—plant-induced oversensitivity to light. This may result in a sunburn soon after eating it—even from being exposed to artificial light. Depending on one's sensitivity and the light intensity, the reaction can range from mild to life-threatening. But just as importantly, in the long-term it contributes to a wide range of symptoms related to actual damage and premature aging of the skin. This includes wrinkles, blotches, spider veins and a loss of skin elasticity. It also predisposes the individual to a significantly higher risk of skin cancer, the so-called photo-carcinogenic effect.

Background

The sun-sensitizing effects of plants of the Apiaceae family were already known to the ancients. Some 4,000 years ago the Egyptians used the juice topically to darken areas of the skin in cases of vitiligo, the gradual loss of skin pigmentation. The Greeks and Romans also learned of these properties. It is still used today as a mainstream therapy for treating this condition, inducing melanin or pigment production in the light-sensitized skin. Celery shares this trait with a number of its family members. Indeed, of all the plants in the world that cause this light sensitivity, fully half belong to the Apiaceae family.

Mechanism

The substances within celery and other members of the plant family responsible for this reaction are called
linear furanocoumarins. These are a type
of *psoralen,* a chemical group found in

Psoralen molecule

a small number of herbs, mostly in the Apiaceae, but also present in members of the Citrus group (Rutaceae). There are other light-sensitizing furanocoumarin chemicals present (bergapten, xanthotoxin and isopimpinellin) that are also well
studied. Because of these substances, celery is the main cause
of phytophotodermatitis reactions. A few other plants, such as
the fig tree, contain these same chemical, but only in the inedible leaves and not in the commonly eaten fruit. The offending
compounds are believed to offer the species some natural pro-
tection against injury from insects, worms and foraging animals. They are also responsible for the microbe-killing properties of celery and other members of the Apiaceae, since they
knock out viruses and fungi through disrupting their DNA
and RNA. Unfortunately, in animals and humans they do the
same, cause death to normal cells (apoptosis). Reacting with
the DNA of the upper layers of the skin, they damage or destroy these tissues. Through the destruction of the epithelial
cells, the deeper layers of the skin are no longer protected
from harmful ultraviolet rays. Oddly, the use of fungicides by
the agriculture industry increases the amount of furanocoumarins in celery. And even organic celery contains pesticides.

Other close Apiaceae cousins of celery also contain furanocoumarins, including parsley, parsnips, lovage, fennel seeds and
carrots. A number of non-edible species, such as *hogweed* and
bishop's weed are well-known as extremely aggressive and toxic

species in this regard. Hogweed will cause burns and blisters through merely touching or brushing up against it and then going out in the sun. Originally from Asia, it has become a persistent weed throughout the Western world. There are laws and regulations in Europe and America to restrict and if possible eradicate this plant entirely. Note that phototoxicity also affects cattle, sheep, white chickens, ducks and pigs, notwithstanding the fact that letting livestock graze on the young plants is one method used to reduce these noxious weeds. The extract from the bishop's weed or lace flower (Ammi majus) is also used, in the correct dose, to make patients intentionally sensitive to ultraviolet therapy for the treatment of psoriasis or the unsightly white patches of vitiligo. In an odd twist, extracts were also used as pigment activators in tanning spas, right up until 1996, with the result of occasional severe burn injuries. Fortunately they are now banned for this purpose.

Source

While the whole plant contains psoralen, it is concentrated in the outer leaves (as appetizing and green as they might look), but also in the mature inner leaves as well. It is present in the root (celeriac) and less so in the stalks. Interestingly, studies showed that celery grown organically or with chemical fertilizers had no effect on the amount of furanocoumarins. But the growing period and climate has an important role.

Exposure

Phytophotodermatitis can occur from ingesting the plant, but also happens from merely handling celery stalks or leaves. Among workers in celery farming and food preparation this takes place with some regularity. But it is also an occupational hazard for grocery store clerks. With the current explosion in sales of the vegetable, there is likely to be an uptick in the number of employees that develop this type of dermatitis, with varying degrees of severity. For consumers handling or juicing celery on a daily basis, such reactions can be expected in a certain percentage of people. Since the content of furanocoumarins present in the plant varies according to the area it was grown, climate and many other factors, it is not possible to determine the risk in advance. Dosage is the key factor, which is also dependent on the affected individual's age, size, weight, skin pigmentation and state of health. Without understanding the possibilities of phytophotosensitivity, consumers may not suspect this hidden cause of a sudden dramatic dermatitis or easy sunburn. Not taking further protective measures for yourself or your family member could make the situation turn quite dangerous.

Effects

A phototoxic reaction can begin in as little as 15 minutes after physical contact or oral ingestion. The effects peak within two hours but can last for days. As mentioned, symptoms range from mild to severe, to extremely serious, just as one would expect with burn trauma. Remember, this is due to the destruction of the upper layer of skin, which itself is both dangerous and painful. Symptoms and signs include swelling, itching, extreme dryness and pain from damage to the rich network of sensory nerves within the dermal layer. There may be typical fluid-filled blisters that can merge to form huge watery masses under the skin (bullae).

Other short-term side effects of psoralen or linear furanocoumarin toxicity include nausea and vomiting and central nervous system (CNS) side effects, including headache, dizziness, depression, insomnia and hyperactivity. Reactivation of cold sores (herpes simplex) is also possible. Because the acute effects of ultraviolet exposure generally last from two to four hours after exposure, merely getting out of the sun does *not* immediately stop the damage to one's skin.

Long-term Effects

A direct result of an Apiaceae burn is local scarring. Over time however, excess ultraviolet damage causes many additional skin aging effects on the exposed areas. This includes darkening (excess pigmentation) or lightening (damage to melanocytes or pigment-producing cells), excess wrinkling, spider veins, brown spots, excess hair growth or even areas of *actinic keratosis*—a precancerous, crusty growth which typically shows up on the hands. Another profound effect is the accumulation of psoralen in the lens of the eye. This results is an increased potential for the development of cataracts.

Down the road there may be an increased chance of skin cancers. As might be expected, people with lighter skin tones are four times as susceptible to psoralen toxins in the generation of melanoma skin cancers, than those with darker skin types. With over two million Americans developing skin cancer every year, an increased risk from celery toxicity should be taken seriously. Oddly, a huge increase in the incidence of cancers of the scrotum or penis has been observed in men from chronic psoralens exposure to *other* parts of the body.

Treatment & Precautions

If you think you may be developing a rash (itching or reddening) from handling or ingesting celery, there are some actions you should take to lessen or prevent further developments.

- If the reaction occurs from handling celery, immediately wash the area with soap and *cold* water.

- Be careful to completely avoid touching the face or eyes.

- Whether due to ingestion or contact, avoid exposure to sunlight for at least 48 hours. Note that this includes light through the windows.

- Both heat and moisture can make the skin reaction worse, so a cool, dry environment is best.

- If it is necessary to go outdoors during the initial time, wear protective clothing, a hat, and use sunscreen.

- Use a natural sunscreen without oxybenzone or other hormone-disrupting chemicals.

For those that have become sensitized by the furanocoumarins of celery, a skin reaction can be triggered by tanning beds or even full-spectrum lighting, which is much stronger in the ultraviolet end of the spectrum. As a preventive, if you have had a reaction (especially in areas where both sunshine and celery sales are prominent) avoid the beach altogether for some weeks.

References

Anaphylaxis Campaign. *Celery Allergy Factsheet* (Dec 2014). Document Reference ACFS1v8© Anaphylaxis Campaign.

Birmingham, D. J., Key, M. M. and Tubich, G. E. (1961). Phototoxic bullae among celery harvesters. *Archives of Dermatology*, *83*(1), 73-87. doi:10.1001/archderm.1961.01580070079008

Diawara, M. M., Trumble, J. T., Quiros, C. F., and Hansen, R. (1995). Implications of distribution of linear furanocoumarins within celery. *Journal of Agriculture and Food Chemistry*,

43(3), 723–727. doi:10.1021/jf00051a030

Furanocoumarins. Retrieved from: https://en.wikipedia.org/w/index.php?title=Furanocoumarin&oldid=883987178"

Nigg, H. N. et al. (1997). Furanocoumarins in Florida Celery Varieties Increased by Fungicide Treatment. *Journal of Agricultural Food Chemistry, 45* (4), pp 1430–1436. doi: 10.1021/jf960537p

Pathak, M. A., Daniels Jr., Farrington; Fitzpatrick, T. B. (1962). The presently known distribution of furocoumarins (psoralens) in plants. *Journal of Investigative Dermatology.* 39(3): 225–239. doi:10.1038/jid.1962.106

Peroutka, R., Schulzová, V., Botek, P. and Hajšlová, J. (2007). Analysis of furanocoumarins in vegetables (Apiaceae) and citrus fruits (Rutaceae). *Journal of the Science of Food and Agriculture, 87*(11), 2152-2163. doi.org/10.1002/jsfa.2979

Seligman, P. J. et al (1987). Phytophotodermatitis from celery among grocery store workers. *Archives of Dermatology* (11):1478 1482. doi:10.1001/arc derm.1987.0166035007-8017

Schulzová, V., Babička, L. and Hajšlová, J. (2012). Furanocoumarins in celeriac from different farming systems: a 3-year study. *Journal of Science of Food and Agriculture, 92*(14), 2849-54. doi: 10.1002/jsfa.5629.

Shenoi, S. D. and Smitha, P. (2014). Photochemotherapy (PUVA) in Psoriasis and Vitiligo. *Indian Journal of Dermatology, Venereology and Leprology.* 80(6) pp497–504. doi:10.4103/0378-6323.144143

Wüthrich, B., Stäger, J., Johansson S. G. (1990).Celery allergy associated with birch and mugwort pollinosis. *Allergy, 45*(8):566-71.DOI: 10.1111/j.1398-9995.1990.tb00941.x

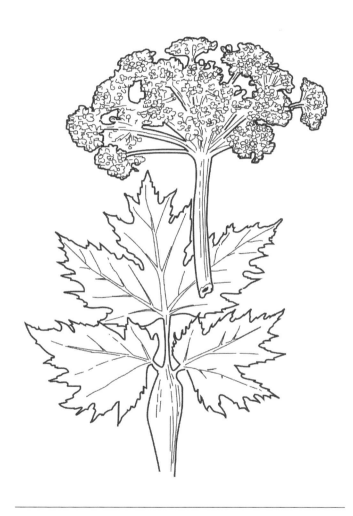

Heracleum maximum - *Giant Hogweed*

3

Suppressed Detoxification

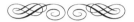

The Facts

One of the most strange notions of the current celery fad is the idea that it is a "detoxifying" agent or part of a detox diet. This is repeated endlessly on blogs, websites and books. Apart from drinking lots of fluid, nothing could be further from the truth. That is because celery belongs to another fairly exclusive group of plants that actually suppress the body's most important form of natural detoxification: the cytochrome P450 system (CYP450). This complex biochemical cleansing process is crucial to every cell in the body. It works to neutralize toxins made in the course of normal biology (endogenous toxins), as well as poisonous substances coming from the environment (exogenous toxins). While there are some 50 enzymes involved in the CYP450 system, studies show that celery significantly blocks at least three of its major components, slowing down or stalling the entire process. Scientists have identified some of the main chemicals that have this effect: imperatorin, trioxsalen, and isopimpinellin, if anyone should ask! To understand the impact of this suppressive effect, we have to look at the way CYP450 functions in the body.

Cellular Effects

■ Along with glutathione, cytochrome P450 is needed for detoxification of the brain, heart, immune system, arteries and all major organ systems.

- It is key to neutralizing a wide range of pollutants, heavy metals, pesticides, plastics and other man-made toxins.

- CYP450 takes part in expelling the remnants of viruses, bacteria, fungi and allergens.

- Environmental carcinogens that the CYP450 system is designed to eliminate are involved with 70% of cancers.

Liver Effects

The liver, being the body's main detoxification organ, is the epicenter of this detoxifying enzyme activity:

- CYP450 is the core of Phase I Liver Detoxification, our first defense to neutralize ingested toxins, food-borne pesticides, additives and so on.

- Phase 2 Liver Detoxification completes the action of converting various chemicals—including alcohol, drugs and various carcinogens—into water-soluble compounds and oxygen.

- It is also needed for creating bile and bile acids that carry off the many toxins that have been chemically bound by the liver. From there, they are deposited into the intestines or circulated to the kidenys elimination.

Biological Effects

The functions of cytochrome P450 actually goes beyond detoxification, playing a major role in overall metabolism. Specifically, it is essential to the body's nutritional status and hormonal balance.

- Bile acids, as mentioned above, are needed for the proper breakdown and absorption of fats and fat-soluble vitamins (A, D, E, essential fatty acids and saturated fatty acids).

- It assists in the creation of vitamin D in the body.

- CYP450 is required for hormone synthesis, in order to create pregnenolone, from which we derive our entire output of estrogens, testosterone and adrenal hormones, such as cortisol and DHEA.

Imagine being on a celery-based detox program that actually suppresses all these functions. This could rightly be called an anti-detoxification diet!

Specific Drug Detox

More than 900 pharmaceutical drugs are potentially toxic to the liver. Numerous drugs also inhibit cytochrome P450 enzymes, making the liver even more vulnerable. Today we are unknowingly ingesting many pharmaceuticals on a daily basis. Indeed, some 69 such compounds have been detected in aquatic ecosystems, and these often work their way up the food chain; Antibiotics are found in milk, cheese and meat; New York tap water contains at least 14 leading pharmaceuticals (including ibuprofen and estrogen); Pollutants in California drinking water could cause more than 15,000 excess cases of cancer according the Environmental Working Group. Since we are under this level of biochemical attack, any suppression of CYP450 through excess celery ingestion can only increase the potential for short and long-term harm from these environment-sourced drugs. The following section will expand on the suppressing effect in relation to specific pharmaceuticals.

Ironically, mainstream medicine has considered using the suppressive ability of celery as therapy. Researchers have suggested that celery extract could reduce smoking, since the nicotene and other addictive substances would be detoxified more slowly and remain in the bloodstream longer. This is probably not the optimal approach to curing addiction.

References

Correia, M. A., and Hollenberg, P. F. (2015). Inhibition of P450 Enzymes in P. R. Oritz de Montellano (Ed.), *Cytochrome P450 Structure, Mechanism, and Biochemistry*, 177-259. Cham, Switzerland: Springer International Publishing.

Deng, X., Pu, Q., Wang, E., and Yu, C. (2016). Celery extract inhibits mouse CYP2A5 and human CYP2A6 activities via different mechanisms. *Oncology Letters, 12*(6), 5309–5314. doi: 10.3892/ol.2016.5317

Gaw, S., Thomas, K. V. and Hutchinson, T. H. (2014). Sources, impacts and trends of pharmaceuticals in the marine and coastal environment. *Philosophical Transactions of the Royal Society of London, 369*. doi: 10.1098/rstb.2013.0572

Jakovljevic, V., Raskovic, A., Popovic, M., and Sabo, J. (2002). The effect of celery and parsley juices on pharmacodynamic activity of drugs involving cytochrome P450 in their metabolism. *European Journal of Drug Metabolism and Pharmacokinetics, 27*(3), 153-156.

Lampe, J. W, et al. (2000). Brassica vegetables increase and apiaceous vegetables decrease cytochrome P450 1A2 activity in humans. *Carcinogenesis, 21*(6), 1157–1162, https://doi.org/10.1093/carcin/21.5.157

4
Drug Interactions

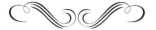

The Facts

Those who have been on prescription medications may have been told by their doctor (or seen it noted on their printed instructions) to avoid eating grapefruit. Celery works in the same way and has an identical prohibition. They both slow the detoxification process, as stated earlier, causing pharmaceuticals to be held in the body for a much longer time. This results in a build-up of the drug, essentially creating an overdose. Depending on the medicine, the resulting side-effects of this excess can vary from mild to life-threatening. Thus celery in any quantity is simply incompatible with a wide range of prescribed medications. Celery also has metabolic and neurological effects that make it unsafe to use when taking the broad range of pharmaceutical drugs that affect the nervous system. Below we list the majority of the known incompatibilities.

Blood Thinners

Celery decreases the body's ability to create blood clots. While this may be desirable in some circumstances, it is contraindicated for those that have bleeding disorders (hemophilia) or are taking medical "blood thinners" for conditions of the heart, arteries or veins, after a stroke and so on. This class of drugs includes common aspirin, heparin, Coumadin (warfarin), Plavix (clopidogrel), Fragmin (dalteparin), Persantine (dipyridamole), Lovenox (enoxaparin), Ticlid (ticlopidine) and others. Taking celery can make the prescribed dosage too high and promote internal bleeding. Also, many nutritionals, such as fish oils (EPA, DHA) have similar blood-thinning properties and will magnify the effect of celery, apart from any pharmaceuticals.

Blood Pressure Medication

Celery can temporarily decrease blood pressure due to its diuretic and artery-relaxing effect. Because of this and the additional slowing of drug detox by the body, it must not be ingested when taking any of the following medications: Captopril (Capoten), enalapril (Vasotec), losartan (Cozaar), valsartan (Diovan), diltiazem (Cardizem), amlodipine (Norvasc), hydrochlorothiazide (Hydrodiuril), furosemide (Lasix) and many others. The increased effect can result in blackouts (syncope) or other drastic or fatal low blood pressure effects.

Anesthesia

It is recommended that all celery use be stopped at least two weeks before general surgery in which anesthetics are used, due to the plant's effects on the nervous system. This makes sense in terms of the widespread neurotoxicity of the compounds in the Apiaceae, epitomized in hemlock (Conium), water hemlock (Cicuta) and dropwort (Oenanthe).

Anti-inflammatory Drugs

Celery prolongs the effect of the common drug acetaminophen (Tylenol) and thus can increase its side effects. Aminopyrine is an example of another anti-inflammatory and anti-fever medicine that requires a healthy liver to be cleared from the body. Because celery can slow the process of breaking down and removing aminopyrine, the direct effects and side effects of these drugs (and most other anti-inflammatory medicines) may be increased.

Anti-thyroid

Celery is known to decrease the effectiveness of thyroid replacement medications, including Synthroid, Armour Thyroid, Eltroxin, Estre, Euthyrox, Levo-T, Levothyroid, Levoxyl and Unithroid.

Lithium

Whether the trace element lithium is being prescribed as a pharmaceutical drug, or taken as a nutritional supplement, celery can interfere with how well the body processes this mineral. That in turn leads to increased levels or overdose, with potentially serious mental and physical consequences, including seizures, coma and death.

Liver-Mediated Drugs

Most drugs must be metabolized by the liver. These include amitriptyline (Elavil), haloperidol (Haldol), ondansetron (Zofran), propranolol (Inderal), theophylline (Theo-Dur and others) and verapamil (Calan, Isoptin). Thus celery can increase the effects—and side-effects—of any of them. Note that the concept of effects and side-effects is strictly in the eye of pharmacological science, not biology. All effects are direct effects, some wanted, some unwanted. This is similar to calling a flower a weed because we don't want it in our garden. Drug effects are a complex matrix of altered body biochemistry and physiology with varying levels of toxicity. A preferred approach is the gentle stimulation of biological repair and regeneration, while removing underlying causes.

Photosensitivity

As discussed earlier, hyper-sensitivity to light can be a serious side effect of celery and other Apiaceae members. But some drugs have the same effect. Anyone on the following medications should avoid using celery in any concentrated dosage. This includes commonly prescribed antibiotics such as Cipro (Ciprofloxacin) and tetracycline, amitriptyline (Elavil), norfloxacin (Noroxin), lomefloxacin (Maxaquin), ofloxacin (Floxin), levofloxacin (Levaquin), sparfloxacin (Zagam), gatifloxacin (Tequin), moxifloxacin (Avelox), trimethoprim/sulfamethoxazole (Septra), methoxsalen (8-methoxypsoralen, 8-MOP, Oxsoralen) and Trioxsalen (Trisoralen).

Sedatives

Sedatives depress or slow various functions of the nervous system. One of the resultant symptoms is drowsiness or sleepiness. Because celery acts similarly, taking them both during the same period of time will increase their "soporific" effects. Sedative drugs in this category include Klonopin (clonazepam), Ativan (lorazepam), Donnatal (phenobarbital), Ambien (zolpidem) and others.

Of course all the above medical drugs have their own extended list of side effects and long-term toxicity. It is important to do personal research on the benefit-risk ratio of any pharmaceutical apart from what is stated on the label or related by your physician, so that an informed decision can be made. Today, the modern medical consumer is able to be far more proactive in participating in their own healing process. However, if the decision is made to take a particular medicine, precautions must be taken. And curtailing celery use is one of them.

References

Jakovljevic, V., Raskovic, A., Popovic, M., Sabo, J. (2002). The effect of celery and parsley juices on pharmacodynamic activity of drugs involving cytochrome P450 in their metabolism. *European Journal of Drug Metabolism and Pharmacokinetics, (27)*, 153–156.

Nguyen, S., Huang, H., Foster, B., Tam, T., Xing, T., Smith, M., Arnason, J., & Akhtar, H. (2014). Antimicrobial and p450 inhibitory properties of common functional foods. *Journal of Pharmacy & Pharmaceutical Sciences, 17*(2), 254-265. https://doi.org/10.18433/J3P599

Rouhi-Boroujeni, H., Rouhi-Boroujeni, H., Heidarian, E., Mohammadizadeh, F., & Rafieian-Kopaei, M. (2015). Herbs with anti-lipid effects and their interactions with statins as a chemical anti- hyperlipidemia group drugs: A systematic review. *ARYA atherosclerosis, 11*(4), 244–251.

5
Nitrites

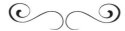

The Facts

Preserving or "curing" meats and vegetables goes back thousands of years, with salt-based dehydration and smoking being the most ancient methods. The purpose of the preservation process is obvious: to destroy the bacteria that would otherwise cause meats, like beef, fish and pork to quickly decompose and become dangerously inedible. Of course the other powerful benefit of food preservation methods is to make various foodstuffs available year round, especially in times of scarcity. But with the advent of modern chemical science and mass production, sodium nitrite and potassium nitrate began to be used as a cheaper and faster (but not more effective) way to create processed meats. Through this method the decay process is greatly slowed, while the animal flesh becomes pink and attractive-looking. This has been the manufacturing standard for the last hundred years, and consumers are likely to be familiar with these additives in luncheon meats, bacon, sausages, salami and hot dogs.

But they also have a bad reputation, going back decades. When combined with red meat under high heat, nitrites form toxic nitrosamine chemicals. This is because, under the effect of heat, they combine with substances found naturally in meats (heme iron, amines and amides) to form carcinogenic and cariodtoxic N-nitroso compounds. This occurs even with small amounts of these chemicals. This has been known for over 40 years, with numerous confirmatory studies. Note that the problem applies to red meat, i.e. pork and beef, but not to white meat, such as chicken and fish.

Nitrate Confusion

So what has this to do with celery? Can't we just avoid these mainstream toxic foodstuffs? This is where things can get confusing. Nitrates occur naturally in many foods, being particularly high in celery. When ingested, they can turn into nitrous oxide (NO), which has many positive effects. In fact, this is one of the factors mentioned by celery promoters as a benefit of high-level consumption. It is also a main reason that another common food—beets—has become popular as a health and energy supplement in recent years.

However, natural food manufacturers have realized that there is strong consumer interest in readily available "no nitrate added" meat products. This sounds attractive to health conscious individuals as an alternative to otherwise carcinogenic meats. But in most cases, what is used as a substitute is our old friend celery powder. It turns out that this has exactly the same effect as chemical nitrates, in use for a century. The result is the production of the same nitrosamines, with the same toxicity, and the same carcinogenic and heart-damaging effects. These are outlined below, with some shocking statistics.

Toxic Effects of Nitrates

- Nitrates and nitrites are linked to an increased risk of cancer, male infertility and early death.

- One sausage or a few slices of bacon daily is enough to raise the likelihood of bowel cancer by 20 percent.

- Eating hot dogs even once a week is associated with higher rates of brain cancer in children.

- The American Institute for Cancer Research advises avoiding processed meats entirely to minimize your risk of bowel cancer, as well as breast cancer.

- After reviewing some 800 studies, the World Health Organization (WHO) classified processed meat as a Group 1 carcinogen, right next to tobacco and asbestos.

- Eating just 9 grams of bacon per day significantly raises a woman's risk for breast cancer later in life.

- Nitrates and nitrites increase the risk of stomach and pancreatic cancer.

- They are associated with an increase in leukemia and brain cancer in children.

- Nitrates are linked to Alzheimer's disease.

- Sodium nitrate contributes to artery damage and hardening of the arteries.

- It interferes with sugar metabolism, increasing the risk of developing type 1 diabetes.

- In infants there is the risk of nitrates causing "blue baby syndrome" or methemoglobinemia by binding with the iron-based protein (hemoglobin) in blood cells. This also occurs from contaminated ground water i.e. well water.

Some of these effects may be due to an excess of saturated fats and toxic compounds produced from cooking these meats. Nevertheless, a major factor is the actual nitrates added to foodstuffs.

Importantly, the old way of curing meats—using regular salt or sodium chloride—has been shown to be equally effective at killing bacteria. It is simply a slower process, and thus not as profitable. In Parma, for example, the local producers stopped using nitrates in their prosciutto back in 1975, opting for the salt-cured method. There has not been a single case of food poisoning and the flavor is said to be greatly enhanced over the standard chemical method.

Adding antioxidants such as vitamin C or vitamin E during processing reduces the toxic effects of nitrates. Similarly, taking a hefty dose of vitamin C (1000 mg) during a meal of these meats will have this preventive effect. Note however that there are many websites, including seemingly credible ones like *Healthlines,* that state that all vegetables contain vitamin C, and thus there is no risk from their nitrate content. This is quite misleading as you will see in Section 4. By looking up the vitamin C content for vegetables on the USDA site or elsewhere, it is clear that some—like celery—have extremely low or even negligible amounts of vitamin C and other common antioxidants. Not all vegetables or herbs are created equal!

An excellent article clarifying the health dangers of bacon, and the obfuscation of the meat industry and governmental agencies, can be found at: https://www.theguardian.com/news/2018/mar/01/bacon-cancer-processed-meats-nitrates-nitrites-sausages

On top of all this, we are under attack from these compounds in drinking water—even many bottled sources. This is because nitrogen-based fertilizers have had a massive impact on nitrate levels in drinking water, especially for the 90% of the US population that still relies on ground water. These high nitrates are directly correlated with N-nitroso in the body (proved through urinary excretion). A number of studies have connected these drinking and well-water levels with increased risk of bladder and ovarian cancers, as well as stomach and brain cancers. Nitrate-contaminated drinking water is also associated with adverse reproductive outcomes (especially neural tube defects), diabetes and thyroid conditions. We certainly do not need additional sources of this chemical, as found in celery powder-based nitrate substitutes.

References

Bahadoran, Z., Ghasemi, A., Mirmiran, P., Azizi, F., & Hadaegh, F. (2016). Nitrate-nitrite-nitrosamines exposure and the risk of type 1 diabetes: A review of current data. *World journal of diabetes, 7*(18), 433–440. doi:10.4239/wjd.v7.i18.433

Etemadi, A., Sinha, R., Ward, M. H., Graubard, B. I., Inoue-Choi, M., Dawsey, S.M. & Abnet, C. C. (2017). Mortality from different causes associated with meat, heme iron, nitrates, and nitrites in the NIH-AARP Diet and Health Study: population based cohort study. *British Medical Journal, 357*(j1957). doi: 10.1136/bmj.j1957.

Mirvish, S. S. (1995). Role of N-nitroso compounds (NOC) and N-nitrosation in etiology of gastric, esophageal, nasopharyngeal and bladder cancer and contribution to cancer of known exposures to NOC. *Cancer Letters, 93*(1), 17-48. doi.org/10.1016/0304-3835(95)03786-V

Ward, M. H. (2009). Too much of a good thing? Nitrate from nitrogen fertilizers and cancer. *Reviews on Environmental Health, 24*(4), 357–363. doi.org/10.1515/REVEH.2009.24.4.357.

6-7-8

Reproductive Health

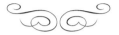

This section brings together several related issues which are brief topics, but with a huge impact. Apart from miscarriage, these issues have not been reported in various news media, blogs, health web pages or medical websites, though the research is readily available. It is not uncommon that investigative reporting falls by the wayside, usually because of the speed in which a trend or fad overwhelms the narrative.

6. Miscarriage

Celery is a traditional and verified abortive agent. It causes uterine contraction and can result in miscarriage or premature labor. In this instance celery seed is particularly at fault, due to its higher concentration of active ingredients like apigenin. This is particularly significant because in the United States, for example, fully 50% of pregnancies are unplanned, representing some 3,000,000 births back in 2013. In fertile women this high celery dosage could certainly be an unidentified cause of miscarriage.

7. Fetal Abnormalities

To quote one source: "Celery extract has abortifacient effects and can cause morphological changes in the embryo, so it is suggested to evaluate the effect of this herb in pregnant women." In animal experiments, the offspring were stunted in height and weight after administration of celery extract to the pregnant mothers. Because of the issue of unexpected pregnancy, celery must be strictly avoided by all women where there is even the remote possibility of pregnancy occurring.

8. Reduced Fertility

Low doses of celery can increase sex hormone production in men and women, but higher doses suppress the creation of estrogen, progesterone and the pituitary hormones that stimulate them: LH (leutenizing hormone) and FSH (follicle-stimulating hormone). Therefore studies show that large amounts of celery definitely inhibit or reduce fertility. These hormonal disruptions have the potential to disturb both a normal pregnancy and the health of the growing fetus.

Other studies have found that celery extract reduces sex hormones overall, affecting the hypothalamus, pituitary and gonads. Some compounds have estrogen-like and anti-androgen (male sex hormone) effects, particularly affecting male sexuality and fertility, while reducing sperm counts. In 2017, an analysis of 16 studies concluded that "Since there are compounds such as apigenin, celery can induce inhibitory effects on fertility in cases of chronic use or high concentration." Celery concentrates has even been used as a traditional method of birth control in India. Thus not only women need to avoid celery, as it contains equal opportunity toxins.

Breastfeeding and Infants

It is recommended that, due to all the known and unknown factors, celery juice should not be consumed by breast-feeding mothers. WebMD states: "There is not enough reliable information about the safety of taking celery oil and seeds in an infant. It is not recommended if you are breast-feeding. Stay on the safe side and avoid use."

That is being rather conservative. With the factors of allergy, photosensitivity, heavy metal toxicity, P450 suppression, neurological effects, and all the issues discussed earlier, it should be avoided by small children altogether.

References

Bonham, A. D. (Oct 21, 2013). Why are 50 percent of pregnancies in the U.S. unplanned? Retrieved from http://shriverreport.org/why-are-50-percent-of-pregnancies-in-the-us-unplanned-adrienne-d-bonham/

Ciganda, C. & Laborde, A. (2003) Herbal Infusions Used for Induced Abortion. *Journal of Toxicology: Clinical Toxicology, (41)*3, 235-239, doi: 10.1081/CLT-120021104

Kooti, W. et al. (2017). The Effect of Celery (Apium graveolens L.) on Fertility: A systematic review. *Journal of Complementary and Integrative Medicine (6)*15. doi: 10.1515/jcim-2016-0141.

Shahedi, A., Kazem, B. S, Mortaza, A., Maryam, Y. and Naeimeh, A. A. (2018). The effect of hydro-alcoholic extract of celery (apium graveolens) leaves on abortion and morphological characteristics of embryo in balb/c mice. *Iranian Journal Of Obstetrics, Gynecology And Infertility, 21* (9), 50-57.

Shinde, P., Patil, P. K., and Bairagi, V. (2012). Herbs in pregnancy and lactation: a review appraisal. *International Journal Of Pharmaceutical Sciences And Research. (12)*9, 3001-3006. doi.org/10.13040 IJPSR.0975-8232.3(9)3001-06

9

Low Blood Pressure

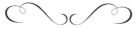

The Facts

Celery does have the effect of causing hypotension (lowered blood pressure). While most people are aware of the frequency of people having hypertension, they might be surprising to learn the large number with blood pressure that is too low. One frequent reason for this is adrenal exhaustion, i.e. burnout from stress. It also occurs in the anemia which is not uncommon in menstruating women. Other typical causes are low blood sugar or hypoglycemia, some heart conditions, diabetes, allergies and even some nutritional deficiencies.

The Complications

Dehydration creates a state of hypotension or low blood pressure. This happens after fluid loss from excess perspiration, fevers, diarrhea and of course hot weather, but is also common in pneumonia and urinary tract infections. Celery is now commonly suggested as a way to hydrate. But since celery is both diuretic *and* blood-pressure lowering, that is definitely contraindicated. It is *not* a preferred method of re-hydrating.

There are also some serious medical conditions where celery juice is not the answer. We can have markedly reduced blood pressure in severe blood loss, trauma, stroke, kidney failure, and the onset of shock (vascular collapse) from any of the above. For those who might consider celery juice a panacea or as part of first aid in any of these conditions, it is once more contraindicated.

I have also read of celery juice being used as a cure or pick-me-up after alcohol use. Alcohol causes a drop in blood pressure generally, so stick to the old tomato juice cure (higher in sodium), as celery will likely makes things worse.

Orthostatic hypotension is that faintness or blacking out feeling that one gets when standing up too quickly. While only about 5% of people have this on a significant level under the age of 50, it is present in 30% of those over 70. As described by Ricci (2015), "It may cause disabling symptoms, faints, and traumatic injuries and substantially reduce quality of life. It "increases mortality and the incidence of myocardial infarction, stroke, heart failure, and atrial fibrillation." Overall, hypotension is a vast subject with copious amounts of scientific studies. Easily overlooked or masked, it is particularly a common risk factor in later age. For all the reasons detailed in this book *the elderly should avoid celery consumption altogether*

References

A decent overview of hypotension can be had on Wikipedia: https://en.wikipedia.org/wiki/Hypotension

Madhavi, D., Kagan, D., Rao, V., and Murray, M.T. (2013). A pilot study to evaluate the antihypertensive effect of a celery extract in mild to moderate hypertensive patients. *Natural Medicine Journal, (5)*4.

Ricci, F., DeCaterina, R. and Fedorowski, A. (2015). Orthostatic hypotension: Epidemiology, prognosis, and treatment. *Journal of the American College of Cardiology, (66)*7, 848-860. doi.org/10.1016/j.jacc.2015.06.1084

10

Bleeding Time

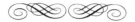

The Facts

Research going back 20 years shows that celery can prolong the time needed for blood to clot, partially by preventing the blood platelets from adhering to each other (platelet aggregation). Celery should be avoided by anyone with a known bleeding disorder (e.g. hemophilia) and individuals taking blood thinners, as mentioned earlier. Symptoms of this clotting deficiency includes easy bruising, pin-point bleeding spots on the legs (petechiae), bleeding gums or nose, or even blood in the urine.

The Double Whammy

While the dose of celery (and the apigenin it contains) that causes this problem is difficult to determine, there is another twist to the story. Many people over 40 take aspirin on the advice of their doctors as a daily blood thinner. Without debating the pros and cons of this regimen, its important to know that aspirin is a major cause of gastrointestinal (stomach and intestine) bleeding. In fact aspirin increases the risk of a bleeding episode by 50%, with 1 in 200 users having a major bleed.

Since aspirin works in the same way as celery, i.e. reducing platelet clumping, the use of celery increases the risk of bleeding in the brain or intestines for those taking aspirin.

References

Medical Press of King's College. (January 22, 2019). *Frequent use of aspirin can lead to increased bleeding.* Retrieved from https://medicalxpress.com/news/2019-01-frequent-aspirin. html

Navarro-Núñez et al. (2008). Apigenin inhibits platelet adhesion and thrombus formation and synergizes with aspirin in the suppression of the arachidonic acid pathway. *Journal of Agriculture and Food Chemistry, 56*(9), 2970-6. doi: 10.1021/jf0723209

Teng, C., Lee, L. G. and Huang, T. F. (1987) *Inhibition of platelet aggregation by apigenin from Apium graveolens.* Retrieved from https://www.researchgate.net/publication/292511412.

US Food and Drug Administration. *Before using aspirin to lower your risk of heart attack or stroke, what you should know.* (Sep 1, 2019). Retrieved from https://www.fda.gov/drugs/safe-daily-use-aspirin/using-aspirin-lower-your-risk-heart-attack-or-stroke-what-you-should-know.

11

Thyroid Disruption

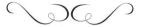

The Facts

Several studies have demonstrated that celery should not be taken in any quantity in those with hyperthyroid disease or with a known celery allergy. Celery has caused actual hyperthyroidism with typical symptoms of blurred vision, palpitation and nausea, sweating and exopthalmos (bulging eyes). And this occurred without any pre-existing thyroid problems. Researchers have suggested that anyone using celery in quantity should have thyroid function tests performed as a precaution. Since celery juice has been used for weight loss, this may be one of the unfortunate mechanisms by which that might occur. This kind of thyroid over-stimulation may have a short-term effect on weight, but is not a solution to hormonal balance or the complex metabolic issues involved with obesity. In fact it is a toxic effect of celery, not a therapeutic benefit.

From a pharmaceutical viewpoint, this may not be seen as a problem, since the accent is on relieving a specific symptom. A drug that kills cancer cells, or that causes sleep, is considered effective even if it does considerable harm to the health of the body overall. Amphetamines, like *Adderall*, do cause weight loss—at great cost. Rarely, such an approach is justified, but getting rid of causative factors is always a better long-term solution than just removing a symptom.

References

Elahe, A., Sadra, A., Mahmoud, R. and Shirin, S. (2017). Effects of substances on plants' active compounds on changes in the hormone levels of the pituitary–thyroid axis in hyperthyroidism and hypothyroidism. *Pharmacognosy Review, 12*(23), 1-6. doi: 10.4103/phrev.phrev_48_17

Kooti, W., Ali-Akbari, S., Asadi-Samani, M., Ghadery, H., and Ashtary-Larky, D. (2015). A review on medicinal plant of Apium graveolens. *Advanced Herbal Medicine, (1)*1, 48–59.

Maljaei, M. B., Moosavian, S, P., Mirmosayyeb, O., Rouhani, M. H., Namjoo, I. and Bahreini, A. (2019). Effect of celery extract on thyroid function; Is herbal therapy safe in obesity? *International Journal of Preventive Medicine 10,* 55. doi: 10.4103/ijpvm.IJPVM_209_17

Rouhi-Boroujeni, H., Hosseini, M., Gharipour, M., Rouhi-Boroujeni, H. (2016). Is herbal therapy safe in obesity? A case of Apium graveolens (celery) induced hyperthyroidism. *ARYA Atherosclerosis,* (12)5, 248–249. doi:10.4103/ijpvm.IJPVM_209_17

12

Kidney Inflammation

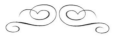

The Facts

In those with any kind of kidney disorder, celery can cause inflammation when used in "medicinal amounts." An 8-ounce glass of celery juice certainly qualifies. It is thought that this is due to the presence of the essential oil (apiole), which is definitely nephrotoxic. That essential oil, extracted from parsley and celery, should only be used externally. It can be fatal if taken internally and deaths have occurred from its use. Paradoxically, several research studies have been done showing celery extract's (apigenin) protective effect on the kidney when powerful anti-cancer and immunosuppressive drugs are used.

References

Blumenthal, M., Busse, W., Golderg, A., Grenwald, J., Hall, T., Riggins, C., et al. (1998). *The complete German commission e monographs: therapeutic guide to herbal medicines.* Austin TX: American Botanical Council.

Brendler, T., Gruenwald, J. and Jaenicke, C. (2007). *PDR for herbal medicines. 4th ed.* Montvale, NJ: Thomson Healthcare Inc.

National Kidney Foundation. (Sep 1, 2019). *Herbal supplements and kidney disease.* Retrieved from https://www.kidney.org/atoz/content/herbalsupp

13

Pesticide Residue

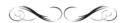

The Facts

Even for those using celery as a reasonable part of their total dietary regimen—or as a specific herbal medicine—there is an added problem. Unfortunately, celery is part of the "dirty dozen" group of plants that carry the largest amount of pesticide residues amongst all fruits or vegetables. In fact, the report by the *Environmental Working Group* put celery at number ten on the no-no list. However, in 2010 it was at the very top of the same list. These reports can be downloaded here: https:// www.ewg.org/foodnews/.

Clearly it is one of the vegetables that should only be purchased organically. This is particularly true for celery seed supplements or extracts. Many spices are also irradiated, further damaging their potential value. However, there is a still a huge problem. To display the USDA organic label, foods only have to be 95% organic. That last 5% can contain about 200 non-organic substances and still have the USDA organic tag. More importantly, even though eating organic significantly reduces how much of top 40 pesticides you are getting, you are still getting them. The Environmental Research report of 2019 measured eight different residues in people's urine, coming from 13 pesticides. After switching to organic, there was a 95% reduction in some residues. But for 5 out of 8, there was only a 40-50% reduction. So the dirty dozen are still dirty, but half as much.

The Toxic Load

Conventional celery contains up to 64 different pesticides as found by the USDA Pesticide Data Program, 95% of all samples testing positive for pesticide residues. These include:

- 10 known or suspected carcinogens
- 27 suspected hormone disruptors
- 12 neurotoxins
- 12 developmental or reproductive toxins

Using products that are properly labeled and verified as organic is the viable choice. But adults and children will still be bombarded by high-pesticide foods.

References

Bienkowski, B. (Mar 20, 2019). *Spinach, strawberries and kale top annual report on the most pesticide-tainted produce.* Retrieved from https://www.ehn.org/fruits-vegetables-with-most-pesticides-2632135188.html

Hylanda, C., Bradmana, A., Geronab, S., R., Pattonc, Zakharevichb, I., Guniera, R. B., & Kleind, K. (2019). Organic diet intervention significantly reduces urinary pesticide levels in U.S. children and adults. *Environmental Research, 171,* 568-575. doi.org/10.1016/j.envres.2019.01.024

USDA Pesticide Database. *Searchable database.* Retrieved from https://apps.ams.usda.gov/pdp.

USDA. *Pesticide residue monitoring 2017 report and data.* Retrieved from https://www.fda.gov/food/pesticides/pesticide-residue-monitoring-program-reports-and-data

What's On My Food. *Celery.* Retrieved from http://www.whatsonmyfood.org/food.jsp?food=CE

14

Heavy Metals

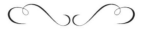

The Facts

One of the most formidable and well-researched challenges to health today is heavy metal toxicity in the form of lead, arsenic, mercury, cadmium, nickel, chromium, aluminum and copper. Some, like mercury and lead, are virulent neurotoxins. Others, like arsenic and cadmium, are known carcinogens. The effects on the immune system, kidney, liver, brain health and quality of life should be on the top of everyone's list of health concerns. Unfortunately the most common way we accumulate these nasty toxins is through food. Heavy metal contamination of the soil is widespread and they are readily absorbed into food crops. Since these toxins stay in the soil, it only worsens over time. Depending on its location, no plant is immune to the bioaccumulation of heavy metals.

Organic Doesn't Help

It is difficult if not impossible to know the origin of most commercially grown vegetables that we purchase. But neither are home gardens immune from heavy metals that have accumulated in the soil for decades. It gets worse, because even if organically grown, vegetables that come to market are not routinely tested for their heavy metal load. After all, It would be both impractical and financially burdensome. Heavy metal contamination has been found in organic baby foods, cat food, children's multivitamins, ginkgo and most other fresh or packaged foods. By the way, this is a global problem, with research showing that cattle in New Zealand, raised for the export of organic meat, had toxic levels of cadmium in their kidneys. In some cases, organically grown products are even more polluted with heavy metals than conventional vegetables. This is because the cow and poultry manure that may have been used as a natural fertilizer is itself highly contaminated with copper, arsenic, cadmium and such. Indeed, one study showed that organic wheat had the same amount of mercury and *twice* the amount of lead as conventional brands.

There are a number of private labs that do test for heavy metals, those of Mike Adams of *Natural News* being at the forefront. But this does not help the average concerned consumer. So what can the average person due to protect themself?

The Heavy Celery Problem

But wait, what has all this to do with the green miracle of celery? It has been found that in a long list of vegetables, the top two plant species that absorb and retain these toxins are *coriander* and *celery*—both members of the Apiaceae family—followed by spinach in third place. In fact a number of studies reveal this same fact. As summarized by one researcher:

> It was also found that celery and parsley leaves have a tendency to assimilate more heavy metals compared to other vegetables.(Glodowska, 2017)

Apart from any other dangers we have written about in this book, this would be a valid reason to not use celery—at all. A useful research project would be testing for lead and other heavy metal concentrations in the blood, hair or other tissues of those on a celery juice program for a number of months.

References

Adams, Mike. *A new standard in food safety.* Retrieved from http://www.lowheavymetalsverified.org/

Dotse, C. K. (2010). Assessing commercial organic and conventionally grown vegetables by monitoring selected heavy metals found in them. *Electronic Theses and Dissertations. Paper 1715.* Retrieved from https://dc.etsu.edu/etd/1715

Głodowska, M. and Krawczyk, J. (2017). Heavy metals concentration in conventionally and organically grown vegetables. *Quality Assurance and Safety of Crops & Foods, 9*(4), 497 - 503. doi.org/10.3920/QAS2017.1089

Kim, H. S., Kim, Y. J., & Seo, Y. R. (2015). An overview of carcinogenic heavy metal: molecular toxicity mechanism and prevention. *Journal of Cancer Prevention, 20*(4), 232–240. doi:10.15430/JCP.2015.20.4.232

Luo, L. et al (2018). Phytoavailability, bioaccumulation, and human health risks of metal(loid) elements in an agroecosystem near a lead-zinc mine. *Environmental Science and Pollution Research Institute, 24,* 24111-24124. doi: 10.1007/s11356-018-2482-4

Hirsch, J. (August 16, 2018). Heavy metals in baby food: what you need to know. *Consumer Reports.* Retrieved from https://www.consumerreports.org/food-safety/heavy-metals-in-baby-food/

McWilliams, J. (Sept 8, 2008). *Rusted Roots.* Retrieved from: https://slate.com/technology/2008/09/is-organic-agriculture-polluting-our-food-with-heavy-metals.html

15
Homeopathy & Microtoxicity

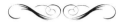

Long Term Effects

Bioenergy medicine is incredibly powerful and does something that pharmaceuticals cannot do: help the body and mind cure chronic disease. But whether you are a homeopathy supporter or a homeopathy denier, the information that follows will be extremely useful, not only in regards to celery, but related to the overuse of any medicine, herb or common food. Even among those who swear by homeopathy's extraordinary 200-year track record of curing everything from allergy to xeroderma, many may not realize its other claim to fame. It is the world's greatest compendium of symptoms and signs arising from the toxicity of plants, minerals and animal substances.

The way homeopathic medicines are researched is by observing the effects of even "normal" substances taken in excess, to discover their long-term effects on *healthy people.* Both subjective and objective symptoms are observed and reported in exquisite detail, with as many test-subjects as possible. Through such studies a picture emerges of symptoms and illnesses produced in every organ system and tissue, in body and in mind. Homeopathic literature—the *Materia Medica*—contains profiles of thousands of such homeopathic medicines. And so it is with celery. Some further explanation is useful in understanding the origin of this comprehensive record of the effects of excess consumption of celery and other medicinal plants.

The Imprinting Effect

The symptoms and disturbances produced during this form of homeopathic research go well beyond the mainstream idea of physical toxicity. They show us that any substance consumed in excess, and for long periods of time, can imprint an individual's biofield, their energetic anatomy. When the information field of a substance is imprinted in this way, its produces its own set of symptoms, superimposed on the individual. Some of these effects are not just temporary, but can last a very long time. Homeopathic doctors call this a *proving* when done in a research setting. If it happens through some type of poisoning or excess ingestion, it is simply an accidental proving. A more meaningful term might be microtoxicity.

Because of this phenomena, symptoms of a proving can be produced in anyone *if a substance is taken frequently and excessively*. Excessive here does not necessarily mean large amounts. Many homeopathic substances are researched using infinitesimal small doses. Some people will always be more susceptible or sensitive than others. But in all cases, if repeated often enough, the substance will produce a set of symptoms that expresses this bioenergetic excess or overdose. The toxic side-effects of drugs are well-known, while mainstream medicine is simply unaware of this imprinting process. However, our physical existence is not based solely on biochemistry, but on complex systems of quantum biophotonic and electrical signaling and information transfer. Repetitive information entrains the body, but excess can become a source of trauma.

In every traditional culture since the beginning of the human journey, diet has varied according to season, cyclic changes and nomadic patterns, so that no food is eaten continually throughout the year. The same applies to the natural diet of mammals, birds and other creatures, and for good reason. If you have been eating or juicing celery in excess, you may have developed any combination of the following symptoms. And if not, it is almost certain that you will after some time!

PHYSICAL SYMPTOMS

The symptoms below are not in anatomical or alphabetical sequence, but more in order of importance and in terms of how disruptive and common they are likely to be.

Headache

- Celery can cause throbbing headaches, focusing on the front or sides of the head, but particularly on the left.
- Like many other symptoms of celery, the pains are worse from movement and from bright light.
- The headache is better from eating something, thus related to disturbances in blood sugar levels.
- The pain is often accompanied by nausea and faintness.
- Throbbing headaches occur that are worse from light or when trying to read.
- During the headache there is restlessness and the inability to sit or lie still.

Insomnia

- Celery can cause an overactive mind and an inability to stop an avalanche of thoughts tumbling over each other.
- This translates into difficulty in falling asleep, due to constant rumination.
- Sleep may also be disturbed by hunger, waking up to eat—yet this doesn't help getting back to sleep.

- Waking between 1 a.m. and 3 a.m. or sleepless till 4 a.m.

- Fidgety legs at night, a form of RLS (restless leg syndrome).

Digestive

- Heartburn, belching and an empty sensation or soreness in the pit of the stomach, somewhat better by eating.

- Loss of appetite in general.

- Diarrhea with pain in the abdomen.

Urinary

- Retention of urine.

Skin

- Urticaria (hives) and itching, with stinging pains that change location, due to either allergy or sun exposure.

- Scratching that causes a change in location of the itch, or creates a burning sensation.

- Red, itchy blotches.

- Itching of the lips.

- Red, elevated pimples as if from the sting of insects.

- A strange shivering or shuddering with the hives or urticaria, that seems unique to celery.

Face

- An odd sensation that the eyes feel drawn in or sunken.

- Itching and burning in the corners of the eyes.

- Sneezing with tickling and running from the nose.

Chest & Lungs

- Shortness of breath; a tickling dry cough; wheezing (these may be asthma-induced symptoms).
- Tightness or intense constriction over the heart region.

Female

- Painful menses, with cutting pain in the region of the ovary, worse with any motion, even by taking a deep breath.
- These cramps are generally relieved by bending forward at the waist (i.e. doubling up).
- Pain in the ovaries and soreness of the nipples.

Joints

- Pains in the neck, together with the low back or sacrum.
- Sacral pain that is better after getting out of bed and moving around, but worse on lying down again.
- Growing pain in the legs, lasting most of the night.

MIND SYMPTOMS

Depression

- Depression is induced, accompanied by feelings of low self-esteem.
- Peculiar feeling that one has said something wrong; the feeling that people tolerate you only to be polite.

Excitability

- Restlessness and constant fidgeting.
- Overexcitability and nervousness.
- Overactive mind, constant thinking. Irritability.

References

Allen, T. F. (1889). *Handbook of Materia Medica and Homeopathic Therapeutics.* Philadelphia, PA: Hahnemann Publishing House.

Clarke, J. H. (1900). *Clarke's Dictionary of the Materia Medica.* London, England: Homeopathic Publishing Company

Clark, B.G. (1922). Apium Graveolens - Celery. *The Homoeopathic Recorder, 37,* 58.

Desai, R. (2005). *Our Magnificent Plants, 2nd Ed.* p290. Kamdern, Germany: Narayana Verlag.

Pelikan, W. The Umbelliferae: Plants of the airy element. (1971). *British Homoeopathic journal, (60)*2, 147-158. https://doi.org/10.1016/S0007-0785(71)80031-5

Pelikan, W. (1971). The Umbelliferae. *British Homoeopathic journal, 60*(3), 194-213. doi.org/10.1016/S0007-0785(71)80053-4

Vermeulen, F. (2003). *Synoptic Materia Medica II.* Apium graveolens. Haarlem, Netherlands: Emryss Publishers.

Wesselhoeft, W.P. (April, 1886). Proving of Apium Graveolens. Ann Arbor, MI: *Medical Advance.*

16

Neurotoxicity

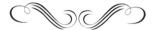

The Theory

This factor is not as deeply investigated as the other, well-researched areas of danger and risk. However, this issue is based on the cumulative evidence coming from a range of evidence. The fact is, the entire family has a powerful relationship to brain function and neurotoxicity. This relates to a series of biochemical substances that are present in the plants. *Polyacetylene* toxins are neurotoxic. *Phthalides* exert powerful effect the brain, but also have toxic effects there. *Apigenin* affects GABA metabolism. We certainly know the added effects of heavy metals and pesticides as hormonal and neurological disruptors. The poisonous factors found in Conium, Cicuta and Oenanthe are found in trace amounts or related compounds in celery. While simple celery can't be called a major neurotoxin, for the many people with various neurological issues, from depression to ADHD, to mania, anxiety disorder, or just overwork and overthinking, it should be used with caution.

Anxiety

The direction that this seems to take is the form of an over anxious, busy and overstimulating mental state. This idea is reinforced by the homeopathic toxicology research, the thyroid-stimulating effect and the traditional description as a stimulant. Overall it is suggested that our phone and internet addicted, adrenalized, caffeinated lives do not need another form of neurostimulation, as the final result is always a weakening of our capacities and biological resources.

References

Burrows, G. E. and Tyrl, R. J. (2013). Apiaceae in *Toxic Plants of North America, 2nd Ed.* (pp 53-58). Ames, IA: Wiley & Sons.

Christensen, L. P. and Brandt, K. (2006). Bioactive polyacetylenes in food plants of the apiaceae family: Occurrence, bioactivity and analysis. *Journal of Pharmaceutical and Biomedical Analysis, 41*(3), 683–693. doi.org/10.1016/j.jpba.2006.01.057.

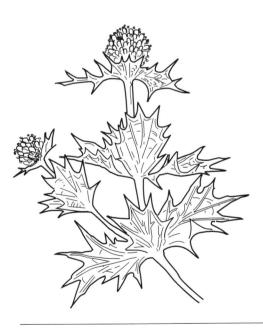

Eryngium maritimum - Sea Holly

Part 3

CELERY TRUTHS & MYTHS

Nutritional Myths

Facts remain facts. But it is possible, without too much trouble, to massage data to look the way one wants. Giving partial information, accenting one idea or omitting other pieces of the mosaic can skew the story in a certain direction. Sometimes this is intentional, sometimes due to negligence, and oftimes just expedient. Journalists, bloggers and health gurus are all very busy and everyone needs fresh new material, new articles and to keep up with the latest trends in the fast-paced news cycle. But when it comes to issues of health, the subject deserves much more caution and investigation.

The Wild Claims

Though you will find literally thousands of identical statements all over the internet and in print, here I quote a well known blog and health information site. In a recent article Natural Health 365 wrote:

> Celery contains many essential vitamins and minerals, such as vitamin C, vitamin K, vitamin A, phosphorus, iron, potassium, magnesium, and calcium.

Dr Axe tells us it is "an excellent source of antioxidants and beneficial enzymes, in addition to vitamins and minerals, such as vitamin K, vitamin C, potassium, folate and vitamin B6."

Selfnutritiondata.com has a complete tables of nutrient amounts found in celery from the USDA, yet in spite of what it shows, the website proclaims "It is also a good source of riboflavin, Vitamin B6, Pantothenic Acid, Calcium."

The Facts

Fortunately, the amounts of nutrients in foods have been studied for many decades and are readily available. The short story is that celery is extremely poor in nutrients altogether, and not "full" of any daily essentials. Note also that the FDA's *recommended daily intake* or RDA for foods remained the same for 50 years. In 2016 there was a revision, and you will find these reflected on food and supplement labels describing the percentage of the RDA that they contain (RDA's are now called RDI's but are essential the same). These numbers are still absurdly low and misleading as they do not take into account physical activity, state of health, environmental risks or a thousand other individual factors. Nor do they reflect clinical or therapeutic amounts, but only what might be needed to keep body and soul together. For example, the RDA for vitamin C has been bumped up to 90 mg, while a good maintenance dose is 1000 mg. In illness, one might need that much per hour. For pantothenic acid (B5), a person may take 500 mg per day for adrenal exhaustion or stress, while the RDA is 5 mg. Whether one wishes to use higher dose nutrients in illness or as a preventive, these RDA figures don't help us understand celery.

By the way, there are actually FDA rules about the words that are commonly tossed about in various claims you may read or hear. There are as follows:

> *"High," "rich in" or "excellent source of" may be used for a food if it contains 20% or more of the RDI. The labels "good source," "contains," or "provides" may be used if it contains between 10% and 20% of the RDI.*

We can see that the amounts required to use these various superlatives are minuscule. In the case of vitamin C, that means that any foodstuff with 18 mg is an excellent source. Possibly a category should be added, stating that if it contains more than the RDI itself, it is "absolutely fabulous!" In any case, such language guidelines are often not followed, and even if they are, the public is highly unlikely to know the rules of the game.

Comparing Apples and Oranges

Most useful is the USDA's (United States Department of Agriculture) full online database, where the nutrient content of common and uncommon foods and food products have been measured and tabulated. There we cab make comparisons can between all these sources. That will give us a measure of how loaded or how impoverished celery is as a food. The information below does not include fruits, nuts, grains, dairy or meats, but is limited to some 768 vegetables (with a few exceptions). Lets see what information we can glean, nutrient by nutrient.

Vitamin C

This top-of-the-list and crucial antioxidant can only be obtained from food (while other animals can manufacture it). How does celery fare? With 3 mg for each 100 g serving, it ranks near the bottom at 642 out of the 763 (bottom 15%). There are very few raw foods in this lowest group, which includes iceberg lecture. Top performers like sweet peppers have a whopping 183 mg, which is a 60-fold increase.

This is not an anomaly, as there are some 75 foods that have over 50 mg per 100g serving—16 times more than celery. And forget about including fruits, such as oranges (144 mg) or kiwis (92 mg). So it is fairly worthless as a source of vitamin C amongst other vegetables. But, if you are stranded on a desert island with no other food, it *might* prevent scurvy.

Vitamin A

Another crucial antioxidant, vitamin A impacts immune function, vision, reproduction, cellular communication, skin, heart, kidneys, the gut lining and more. While it is a fat-soluble nutrient, it is found in many plant species. And celery? It is in the middle of the pack, half way down, with 26 mg per 100 g serving. A sweet potato has well over 900 mg, 30 times better, and there are over a hundred vegetables that have 300 mg and above. Celery is of minimal value as a source of vitamin A.

Beta Carotene

The carotenoid that your body can turn into vitamin A gives carrots their bright color. But it is not uncommon to find people who genetically cannot make this transformation, and must rely on dietary vitamin A. The carrots we mentioned carry a whopping 8300 mcg, while celery has 270 mcg per 100g, exactly half way in a list of 540 vegetable-based foods. Watercress or bib lettuce gives you 1900 mg, while winter squash give you 10 times (1000%) the amount in celery . Not a useful source.

Lutein

One of the very important carotenoids, lutein is rightly famous for being the antioxidant protecting the retina and preventing macular degeneration and cataract. But current research also shows that it is prominent in various regions of geriatric brain tissue and that supplements will improve cognition and brain function. Celery is again a mid-range source, with 200 other vegetables ahead of it in content. With only .28 mg per 100 g, try spinach, kale or chard with a phenomenal 10-15 mg, about 14 times as much. And in the USDA's list of recommended foods rich in lutein, celery is nowhere to be found.

Vitamin K

Essential for blood clotting and calcium metabolism, vitamin K (phylloquinone) can be had from food or made in the colon (menaquinone). But supplement sources are important. Celery moves up to the upper third, with 30 mcg. Still, there are 180 foods ahead of it, far exceeded by vegetables like asparagus (80 mcg), spinach (483 mcg) and Swiss chard (800 mcg). As a vegetable it is not a key source of vitamin K.

B Vitamins

Since we have recurrent statements of celery being a rich source of the eight B vitamins, here is a brief fact-check of a few of these vital nutrients: B6 (pyridoxine), B5 (pantothenic acid) and B2 (riboflavin). Again, the RDI of B vitamins is quite low, compared to B supplements, which may contain 50 or 100 mg.

B5 (pantothenic acid) comes in at .25 mg per 100 g of celery, while we need 10 mg per day. It is in the middle of the pack, around the same as beet greens, corn and many others, meaning there are 300 better vegetable sources. But stepping outside of the realm of vegetables, we have egg yolks, having 12 times as much, and good old brown rice, with 600% more B5.

B6 (pyridoxine) has a wide range of functions, but its role in the production of brain chemicals like serotonin and melatonin stand out. Celery contains .074 mg per 100g, putting it in the bottom 25% of vegetables. Garlic has 1600% more, but even a baked potato offers 9 times as much.

B2 (riboflavin) plays a key role in energy metabolism. It weighs in at .057 mg per 100 mg. Spinach has four times as much and mushrooms 7-8 times the concentration. Of course you could use marmite (yeast spread) and get 300 times the amount.

Folic Acid is an essential B vitamin that must be mentioned since countless websites, including the prominent *www.thetruthaboutcancer.com* declares that celery is "naturally rich in vitamins and minerals such as A, C, K and folate." We know the first three are not, so what about folate? In 100 g of celery there are 36 mcg, which is only 1/10th of the RDA of 400 mcg, while supplements usually contain 800 mcg. Leeks and soy beans have 10 times more. Spinach, seaweed and asparagus and many others have close to 200 mcg .Sunflowers seeds have 240 mcg, around the same as a same small portion of beef or chicken. To put that in perspective, a chicken breast is about 200 g, so your RDA of 400 mcg is covered right there, without the problems associated with celery. All in all, celery is well below average even amongst its peers in the leafy plant world. It is simply a very poor (not a "naturally rich") source of B vitamins overall.

Calcium

There are also consistent claims of the high mineral content of celery, citing calcium, magnesium, potassium, sodium and others. Chopped celery turns in at 40 mg, while kale has 700% more. Still, it is in the middle of the 500 vegetable products, so there is something there, but hardly stellar or a main source from the vegetal world. Without unfairly bringing in cheese (approximately 1000 mg), sesame seeds also have 2500% more (960 mg) and almonds turn in a decent 350 mg.

Magnesium

Celery fares far less well with magnesium, which is possibly the most common mineral deficiency, at a paltry 11 mg per 110 g down in the bottom 13% of sources. Try shiitake mushrooms with 132 mg (1200% more), or sun-dried tomatoes with 194 mg. But there are hundreds of other choices.

Zinc

It gets worse. Zinc is an essential trace mineral that is involved with hundreds of body processes: immune function, protein synthesis, DNA synthesis, cell division, normal taste and smell and more. The FDA recommends 10 mg a day, while supplements contain 30 mg. A cup of oysters gives you 74 mg, cremini mushrooms, just 1 mg. But the zinc content of celery is trace, with only .13 mg, in the bottom 7% of all vegetable sources.

Potassium

Surely potassium will save the day, since celery is a "rich source." It does rise to the occasion, but not far, being in the very center of 760 vegetable sources. Beet greens are victorious with 762 mg. Celery has a third of that at 260 mg, with baked potato at 572 mg and spinach at 558 mg. But if you need a potassium boost, a medium-sized banana contains 420 mg.

Iron

The main source of iron for many people is beef, chicken, seafood and other forms of heme iron, that are more absorbable than plant sources. Still, while a serving of 100g of beef might give you 6 mg of iron, spirulina has a significant 28 mg. In the bottom 2% of all vegetables, celery has a minute .2 mg.

So why are so many promoting the complete myth that this nutrient-poor and mineral-poor plant is so loaded with goodness? Yes, you can take massive amounts to increase the level of nutrients, but you could do the same with any food. And then you are also significantly increasing all of celery's risk factors and side effects of psoralens, apigenin, heavy metals, pesticides, detox suppression, light sensitivity, allergenicity, nitrites, infertility, bleeding and so on.

Sodium

Finally we come to sodium, which is generally in excess in the average Western diet:

> A deficiency of sodium does not occur under normal conditions even with diets very low in sodium. In contrast, an excess of sodium in food is common to most populations worldwide. (Strazullo, 2014)

Fortunately celery is just a fair source at 80 mg per 100 g with 300 higher vegetable sources. In this case its deficiency in nutrients has a benefit, as otherwise there would be far more drastic results from consuming excess amounts of the plant. The potassium to sodium ratio is about 3:1, which also helps it from being too overwhelming. Of course, there is nothing special about this sodium, no magical properties whatsoever.

As the main cation in the body, sodium relates to permeability of cell walls, blood and fluid volume, nerve conduction and heart activity, to name a few core functions. It is simply a crucial electrolyte, governing fluid movement in and outside the cell. But it has nothing directly to do with the process of detoxification. For that, the body relies on the P450 system and sophisticated processes with names like sulfonation, glucoronidation and methylation to clear toxins from the tissues and allow them to become water soluble and be easily excreted. Liver, skin, lungs, kidneys, intestines and colon are all part of these extraordinary cleansing pathways of the organism. That is quite distinct from sodium's vital functions. This is mentioned solely because of claims that sodium in celery pulls toxins out of the body, creates HCl and other phantasmagorical ideas. But if one wants to delve into the real esoteric aspects of minerals, Pelikan's "Secrets of Metals" is a fascinating read.

Celery is Not a Food!

Going back to the original premise of this book, celery is a medicine. It is an herbal drug that has been ported over into the food category and used as an occasional addition to our culinary life. The real effects of celery come not from its nutritive ability, but its active medicinal substances. It is not a regenerator and does not contain a spectrum of nutrients to build or maintain a healthy body or mind. This is also where the understanding that medicines are dose-dependent comes into play.

Indeed there are one or two compounds in celery that may have a unique role, once well researched. The vast majority of its medical uses however, and the biochemical substances responsible for them, are by no means exclusive to this plant. For most of celery's medical effects there are dozens and sometimes hundreds of plants doing a better job, and with less toxicity or risk. It is not the purpose of this brief book to examine each and every one of these substances and each biological effect, but we can hit some of the high points in the next chapter.

References

Heiting, Gary. (December, 2017). *Lutein and zeaxanthin: Eye and vision benefits.* https://www.allaboutvision.com/nutrition/lutein.htm

Nutrition Data. Retrieved from https://nutritiondata.self.com/facts/vegetables-and-vegetable-products/2396/2

Pelikan, W. *Secrets of Metals* (1973). Herndon, VA: Lindisfarne Books.

Strazzullo, P., & Leclercq, C. (2014). Sodium. *Advances in Nutrition, 5*(2), 188–190. doi:10.3945/an.113.005215

Swanson, A (May 10, 2018. *The fda's new recommended daily intake for multivitamin labels: Why the change?* Retrieved from: https://thehealthbeat.com/the-fdas-new-recommended-daily-intake-for-multivitamin-labels-why-the-change

USDA Food Composition Databases. Retrieved from https://ndb.nal.usda.gov/ndb/nutrients/index?fg=13&fg=9&nutrient1=303&nutrient2=&nutrient3=&subset=0&sort=c&totCount=0&offset=0&measureby=g

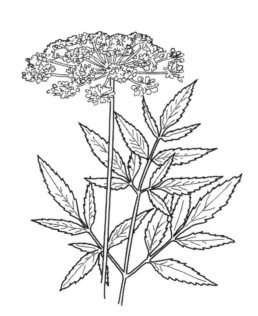

Cicuta virosa - *Water Hemlock*

Benefits & Caveats

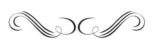

A Treasury of Plant Medicines

There is a lot of plant healing available out there. An estimated 4 billion people rely on plants as their sole source of medicine. Yet only 15% of the 250,000 species of plants on the planet have been scientifically screened for their healing potential. For example the National Cancer Institute (NCI) studied about 35,000 random plant species for anticancer activity over a 20 year period— yielding two useful drugs. Nonetheless, there is an incredible treasure trove of herbal medicines in the traditions of Europe, India, China and the Americas. Even some of the most poisonous plants have given us remarkable medicines, and for the last quarter of a century, 25% of all prescriptions in the US were plant-derived. The drug L-dopa, used in Parkinson's, is extracted from the horny goat weed plant, while Tamoxifen, a synthetic form of the chemical found in the Pacific yew tree (Taxus brevifolia) treats cancer through hormonal suppression. Sometimes these isolated bioactive principles are the most beneficial. In other contexts, the whole plant is still the best therapeutic choice.

Modern pharmacology has taken a renewed interest in indigenous and botanical medicines as a safer alternative to chemicals cooked up in the laboratory. Still, the medical approach is to find the active ingredients or biochemical component that can be isolated, extracted—or synthesized. This is not only to make the resultant drug more potent and the dosage measurable. It means it can be produced in quantity, as opposed to extracting it from tons of raw plant. And there is the possibility

to patent these chemicals for a massive profit. The most famous—and the first of these—is aspirin (acetylsalicylic acid),
found naturally in willow bark. In general, the use of a whole
plant with its complementary nutrients and co-factors is preferable, but not always possible. Hyoscyamus (henbane) yields
the anti-nausea drug scopolimine. But as an herb it is a wild
hallucinogen that can produce death through seizures. All
this is to say that celery is a small player in a vast sea of botanical medicines. It has value, but in its proper perspective.

Biochemical Complexity

To discuss or debate the findings of hundreds of studies of celery, or any of the scores of substances found in the Apiaceae,
would require several textbooks. Here we will just mention a
few of the stated benefits, and try to understand what is really
going on, and if virtue lies beneath overblown claims. For
those who want to delve deeply into the complexities and jar-
gon of biochemical research, there are some excellent resources. For a comprehensive profile of *Apium graveolens* from a therapeutic, biochemical and botanical perspective Jillian Stansbury's extensive review, or the comprehensive paper by Kooti
are excellent resources listed in the references below. There
one can find detailed information about the benefits of this
plant as a modern medicine. But you will not get those benefits, and instead many of the downsides, from drinking huge
amounts of celery juice daily. The majority of the research related to celery has been done using specific bioactive ingredients, not the whole plant. Or the celery concentrate is injected
into an area of the test animal. But before looking at specific
celery effects, there are some general concepts about research
that need to be examined.

Animal Studies

The ethics of using animals in drug and medical research is a controversial issue (and I fall on the "don't do it in the current way" side of the argument). But that aside, it is old news that animal studies do not accurately predict effects on human beings. Most celery studies have been carried out with laboratory rats, including those testing the ability to protect the liver (hepatoprotection) or kill cancer cells (cytotoxicity).

First of all, "mice are not furry little people" as NPR's 2017 article states. Their metabolism, biochemistry and reactions have similarities to human beings, but there are also very significant differences (apart from size). A number of scientists feel that this is the reason why so many pharmaceutical drug trails fail when they get to the human phase, after showing some success in a rodent study. In fact less than 10% show benefit and reach the approval level. Even then, this long drawn-out research often fails. An astounding 32% of FDA approved drugs have unforeseen problems after being on the market. There is great financial pressure and momentum to still do things the old way. And thus the very first thing to look at in any promising celery study is if, at least, there are results of human studies. Secondly, examine the risk and potential toxic effects.

Misinterpreting Science

Scientific research collects observations and facts. But unfortunately research data can be massaged in all kinds of ways, some of them misleading. A recent article from a reputable online health information resource proves the point. *Luteolin* (LU) is a flavonoid found in more than 300 plant species, many readily available in the human diet. Recently it has been shown to have potential in cancer treatment. The headline at Green-

MedInfo.com reads "Celery compound may halt HRT breast cancers." In this article the research study is reported and celery is mentioned as the first of a short list of foods containing luteolin. But a simple check of the USDA list of flavonoids in some 307 foods finds that oregano contains *over 1000 mg of luteolin* per 100 grams of the food. Meanwhile, fresh celery has only *4 mg per 100 g!* Celery is also significantly beaten out in luteolin content by olives, thistles, artichokes, lettuce, bell peppers and many others, and has about the same amount as broccoli or lemons. Yet celery is the entire focus of the article. It is very easy to tweak scientific data in a specific direction to support a fad, current trend or just to create a newsworthy blog post. (http://www.greenmedinfo.com/blog/celery-compound-may-halt-hrt-breast-cancers February 4th 2017)

As with any medicine (not food), taking celery in high dosages is a matter of benefit-risk ratio. Because of this, looking at the effects of one isolated biochemical ingredient found in celery is of limited value. The concentration of such substances can be minute, and in order to have an effect, celery (or any other plant) would have to be taken in abnormally large amounts or concentrations. Again, this is the difference between foods and medicines. The best eating practice in general is to use a wide variety and range of vegetables in salads, soups or side dishes. It makes perfect sense that our bodies evolved to enjoy different colors, flavors and textures in our plant-based foods. Apart from their visual or gustatory value, their differences are a result of the vast number and complex combinations of phytochemicals, bioflavonoids and nutraceuticals. All living creatures seek that variety as part of the body's biological wisdom. With these caveats, we can look at some of the scientific highlights relevant to using celery as a concentrated medicine.

References

Chen, C. *FDA increasingly approves drugs without conclusive proof they work.* (Jun 26, 2018). Retrieved from: https://www.pbs.org/newshour/health/fda-increasingly-approves-drugs-without-conclusive-proof-they-work

Bracken M. B. (2009). Why animal studies are often poor predictors of human reactions to exposure. *Journal of the Royal Society of Medicine, 102*(3), 120–122. doi:10.1258/jrsm.2008.08k033

Downing N. S. et al. (2017). Postmarket safety events among novel therapeutics approved by the us food and drug administration between 2001 and 2010. *JAMA (317)*18, 1854-1863. doi: 10.1001/jama.2017.5150.

Giles, J. 14 December 2006. Animal studies: a good guide for clinical trials? *Nature Magazine.* doi:10.1038/news061211-15

Katiyar, C., Gupta, A., Kanjilal, S., & Katiyar, S. (2012). Drug discovery from plant sources: An integrated approach. *Ayu.* 33(1), 10–19. doi: 10.4103/0974-8520.100295

Kooti, W., and Daraei, N. (2017). A review of the Antioxidant activity of celery (Apium graveolens L). *Journal of Evidence-Based Complementary & Alternative Medicine, 22*(4), 1029–1034. doi:10.1177/2156587217717415

NPR. (April 10, 2017). Drugs that work in mice often fail when tried in people. Retrieved from https://www.npr.org/sections/health-shots/2017/04/10/522775456/drugs-that-work-in-mice-often-fail-when-tried-in-people

Stansbury, J.(Mar 21, 2016). *The apiaceae family – medicinal plant research summary.* Retrieved from: http://battlegroundhealingarts.com/articles/the-apiaceae-family-medicinal-plant-research-summary/

ANTI-MICROBIAL ACTION

Biochemical extracts from celery have been used in blood products (for transfusion) to kill off any viruses present. But its use as a human antiviral is a bad idea. There are scores of powerful and non-toxic anti-virals in the herbal realm. My favorite is olive leaf extract, which is almost infallible for common viral infections. Add to this an effective nutritional supplement like reduced glutathione and you have an antiviral cocktail that also improves cellular metabolism and detoxification. The anti-microbial effects of celery are due to one of its toxic properties—psoralens—and so the risk-benefit ratio is questionable. An ideal antimicrobial should be specific enough to kill viruses or fungi without toxic damage to our own cells.

References

Gautam, P. (2013). Antiviral potential of medicinal plants: an overview. International *Research Journal of Pharmacy, 4*(6), 8-16. doi: 10.7897/2230-8407.04603

Lin, L., Hsu, W. and Lin, C. (2014). Antiviral natural products and herbal medicines. *Journal of Traditional and Complementary Medicine, 4*(1), 24-35. doi.org/10.4103/2225-4110.124335

Redfield, D. C., Richman, D.D., Oxman, M. N. and Kronenberg, L. H. (1981). Psoralen inactivation of influenza and herpes simplex viruses and of virus-infected cells. *Infection and Immunity, 32*(3), 1216-26.

Blood Pressure

The blood pressure lowering action of celery in rats is caused by *vasodilation*. This muscle-relaxing effect on blood vessels seems to be through a calcium-channel-blocking effect. Thus it will have the same toxic impact as typical calcium-channel blocking drugs. There are at least a dozen such drugs (i.e. Norvasc) with a long list of potential side effects, including constipation, headache, palpitations, dizziness, rashes, drowsiness, flushing, nausea and swelling in the feet and lower legs. Blood pressure can be lowered by throwing off large amounts of urine through celery's diuretic effect. This is a further confirmation that celery is a medicine being used as a vegetable, not the other way around. Neither of its effects corrects the causes of hypertension: It is symptomatic only. There are far better choices in the herbal and nutritional field that can address deeper issues and causative factors, without toxicity.

Blood Sugar

In one study of 16 prediabetics, blood sugar was lowered, but with no effect on insulin—insulin deficiency being the mechanism of diabetes. So we don't really know what is taking place, or if this effect is a toxic by-product. Fixing the pancreas, liver, adrenals and organs involved with starch and sugar metabolism is preferable to merely producing a symptom change.

References

Yusni, Y., Zufry, H., Meutia, F. and Sucipto, K. W. (2018). The effects of celery leaf (apium graveolens L.) treatment on blood glucose and insulin levels in elderly pre-diabetics. *Saudi Medical Journal.* 39(2),154-160.

BRAIN CONDITIONS

The most promising medicine that may emerge from the humble celery is an ingredient called 3-nbutylphthalide or 3nb. Butylphthalide is largely responsible for the taste of celery. It is probably the chemical that affects high blood pressure, both as a diuretic and through relaxing the blood vessels. Dr. Murray mentions that it acts like typical medical drugs in these regards, but with the benefit of not disturbing the sodium-potassium ratio of the blood, nor reducing blood from to the brain. Like ginkgo, it increases brain blood flow.

The 3nb extract was approved in China for the treatment of cerebral ischemia (lack of oxygen due to reduced blood flow). It appears to be beneficial for those who have suffered a stroke or other brain injury. This is where symptomatic treatment shines—in acute emergency or trauma. If someone just had a stroke, we are not worried about modifying diets or unhealthy lifestyles, or even the decades of contributory toxins. We want that person to survive and recover. After weeks or months of rehabilitation, diet and nutrition can take a more prominent role. As a longer term effect, in mice that have a chemically induced Parkinson's disease (destroying the dopamine-producing part of the brain) 3nb showed a neuroprotective, antioxidant effect, increasing the dopamine-producing neurons.

Indeed, an extract of celery seed with 85% 3-n-butylphthalide (about 65 mg) is now readily available from a number of vitamin manufacturers. It is fascinating that, with the powerful neurotoxins and neuromodulators in the Apiaceae family, its greatest therapeutic value may be in how it affects the brain itself. But even in this case, gallons of celery juice will not provide this benefit in enough concentration, without the chain of other negative effects discussed throughout this book.

References

Chen, Y et al. (2019). Dl-3-n-butylphthalide exerts dopaminergic neuroprotection through inhibition of neuroinflammation. *Frontiers of Aging Neuroscience.* doi.org/10.3389/fnagi.2019.00044

Lin. G. et al. (2005). Chemistry and biological activities of naturally occurring phthalides. *Studies in Natural Products Chemistry 32,* 611-669. doi: 10.1016/S1572-5995(05)80065-1

Murray, M. (2019, Sep 1). *Celery and celery seed extract are powerful-proven healers.* Retrieved from https://doctormurray.com/celery-and-celery-seed-extract-are-powerful-proven-healers/

Xue, L. X., et al (2016). Efficacy and safety comparison of DL-3-n-butylphthalide and Cerebrolysin: Effects on neurological and behavioral outcomes in acute ischemic stroke. *Experimental and Therapeutic Medicine, 11*(5), 015–2020. doi:10.3892/etm.2016.3139

CANCER

Talk of the "big C" immediately strikes fear into the heart, and can be used in all kinds of persuasive and misleading promotions. Cancer is a huge topic, as is the holistic approach to this condition. And there are mistakes on both sides of the fence. First, cancer is not "cured" solely by killing off cancer cells. Not until causative factors, tendencies, and susceptibilities are removed, and the body's defenses optimized, can there be a well-defined cure. Sometimes the cancer killing regimen can kill the patient much faster than the disease, as was the case with my mother. On the other hand, thinking that someone with invasive tumors and a very weakened immune system can shrink their cancer with natural products is a huge "ask." It is possible, but very unlikely that the body has the inner resources to respond to these natural promptings. There is a balance required. We can eliminate tumor tissue and minimize potentially lethal and damaging therapies as much as possible. At the same time we can use the broad resources of food, supplements, herbs and homeopathics to our advantage.

The field of *bioactive foods* and *nutraceuticals* for cancer prevention is already quite vast, and going strong for decades, with a library of books and research papers showing the healing power of every kind of foodstuff. For example, there are hundreds of studies of the mustard plant family—cabbage, kale, Brussels sprouts, broccoli, etc. and their load of cancer-preventing glucosinolates and indoles. You can even buy these easily as vitamin concentrates. The ferritin in milk is a powerful anti-cancer agent. Pomegranate for prostate cancer, green tea preventing lung cancer, apples for colon cancer, turmeric for stomach cancers, raspberries in throat cancer, cinnamon for a variety of cancer tumors, artichokes for skin cancer—the list goes on and on. An internet search will reveal many of the top 20 or 30 cancer-preventing foods, in which celery is notably absent. In the scheme of bioactive foods it is a player, but a minor one, with a number of toxic drawbacks.

Here we have not mentioned the known anti-cancer effects of hundreds of botanical herbs and well known nutrients. There is an entire field of study focusing on thousands of bioactive substances in medicinal plants, as applied to disease and disease prevention. And there are hundreds of effects, with names like chemoprotective (protecting from chemicals), antiproliferative (stopping excess cell production), antigenotoxic (protecting the DNA), etc. Without appreciating the extent of this field of study and application, it is easy to make a fuss over the fact that this lone vegetable, celery, may have a cancer preventive effect. More specifically, there are 4 factors in celery touted as anti-cancer:

Luteolin: As mentioned earlier, this flavonoid is very common in the plant world, celery being low on the list of sources.

Apigenin: While there is some anti-cancer effects, basically apigenin kills cells (i.e. cytotoxic). It is a fascinating substance with many effects. Chamomile tea is a far richer source. However, it also does hurt the liver (hepatotoxic) and is genotoxic (damages DNA).

Falcarinol: This chemical seems to act against cancer cells in the colon, but is actually found in high concentration in carrots, not celery. It is also toxic in large enough amounts.

Furanocoumarins. Recall these compounds that can destroy the upper layer of skin cells and thus cause photosensitivity? Due to their toxicity, they can also destroy cancer cells.

There are compounds that help the body's process of destroying or suppressing cancerous cells, and there are also chemicals that are extremely poisonous and just kill cancer cells more easily than regular cells. The line between these two kinds of compounds is not always clear. Obviously it is preferable to use less toxic materials to get the same job done.

References

Eisenbrand, G (Ed.) (2000). *Carcinogenic and anticarcinogenic factors in food symposium.* Weinheim, Germany: Wiley-VCH Verlag.

Hsieh, C. C., de Moura Bell, J. and Hernandez-Ledesma, B.(Eds.). (2015). *Food bioactive compounds against diseases of the 21st century.* London, England: Hindawi Publishing Corporation. doi.org/10.1155/2015/241014

Mine, Y. et al (Ed.). (2011). *Bioactive proteins and peptides as functional foods and nutraceuticals.* Ames, IA: Wiley-Blackwell.

Singh, P., Mishra, S. K., Noel, S., Sharma, S. and Rath, S. K. (2012). Acute exposure of apigenin induces hepatotoxicity in Swiss mice. *PloS one, 7*(2), e31964. doi:10.1371/journal.pone.0031964

Toxicology Data Network. *Apigenin.* https://toxnet.nlm.nih.gov/cgi-bin/sis/search/a?dbs+hsdb:@term+@DOCNO+7573

Watson, R. & Preedy, V. R. (Eds.). (2011) *Bioactive foods and extracts: cancer treatment and prevention.* Boca Raton, FL: CRC Press.

CHOLESTEROL

Rats that are bred to have high cholesterol benefited from injections of celery extract, though according to researchers, the mechanism is unknown. But we do know that it is not through reducing the excess production of cholesterol or its causes, but by making the body excrete it more readily. Interestingly in these experiments the triglycerides became higher in the liver, due to suppression of the P450 system. There are natural ways to reduce cholesterol without celery's risks, including flax seed, garlic, adzuki beans, oats (fiber), pectin-containing fruits like apples, fish oils and so on. An isolated effect like this is at the core of drug research, not health research, and does not translate into taking celery as a medicine, or a staple food.

DETOXIFICATION

Mannitol, the kind of sugar that is found in particularly large amounts in celery, can cause bloating and diarrhea. This is not detoxification. Purging the bowels may have its uses, but in this case the reaction is not the process of getting rid of toxins in general. It is because mannitol itself is acting as a toxin. That is exactly what the body is getting rid of, while losing valuable fluids, minerals, amino acids and upsetting the intestinal flora or biome. Differentiating between a healing process (or crisis) versus a toxic reaction or disease progression is a huge topic. But suffice to say there are very well-defined indicators.

References

Tsi, D., Das. N. P. & Tan, B. K. (1995). Effects of aqueous celery (Apium graveolens) extract on lipid parameters of rats fed a high fat diet. *Planta Medica. 61*(1), 18-21. doi: 10.1055/s-2006-957990

LIVER FUNCTION

In herbal medicine, a plant that stimulates bile production from the liver, or causes the gall bladder to release its store of bile, is called a *cholagogue*. There are numerous herbs with this effect. A typical list, from the P.C.C.E. (pre-celery-craze-era) lists 17 well-used herbs, including aloe, barberry, burdock, dandelion, gentian, ginger, goldenseal, milk thistle, peppermint and turmeric. Similarly an excellent summary paper by the College of Integrative Medicine gives us an overview of some 30 prominent cholagogues, choloretics, hepatics, hepatoprotectives and hepatorestoratives, that have both a long traditional history and adequate clinical and laboratory research behind them. Understandably, celery is nowhere on these lists. Saying that celery "rebuilds the bile" is nonsensical.

References

Lloyd, I. (Ed). (2019, Sep 1). *Cholagogue* in ND Health Facts. Retrieved from http://www.ndhealthfacts.org/wiki/Cholagogue

Sodano, W. L. (2015). *Herbal medicine approach to hepatobiliary dysfunction.* College of Integrative Medicine: Hampstead, MD. Retrieved from https://www.collegeofintegrativemed-

icine.org/uploads/filemanager/source/Herbal%20Medi-
cine%20for%20Hepatobiliary%20Dysfunction_1.pdf

MALE FERTILITY

A rat study showed that celery leaf extract may improve sperm
production and increase the size of the testes and tubules,
such that it might be useful for sperm fertility in humans. The
mechanism for this effect is unknown. However, as previously
mentioned research points out, this is dependent on dose.
Smaller doses stimulate, and higher doses suppress hormone
production. You could say this is a homeopathic type of effect

STOMACH ACID

Hydrochloric acid (HCl) deficiency is very widespread, particularly past middle age. Without adequate HCl there is likely to
be malabsorption of calcium, iron and protein — the three nutrients that are most typically deficient in the elderly. This is
largely due to atrophy of the stomach lining and long term
damage to the cells that produce it, the so-called *chief cells*.

The tradition of using of herbal "bitters" to stimulate digestion (HCl production) goes back thousands of years. Many of
these have been scientifically verified. Formerly a popular be-
fore-dinner aperitif in Europe, these are now readily available
as herbal combinations that include dandelion, gentian, arti-
choke, burdock, yellow dock or barberry. To this might be added warming *carminatives* like ginger, pepper or cinnamon.

One can also take an HCl replacement, i.e. betaine HCl, made
from beets, which also stimulates the function of our own ac-
id-making cells. Probiotic-containing fermented foods are
helpful and apple cider vinegar is can be strikingly effective.

Celery contains some bitter principles that could have an effect, but animal studies demonstrate that *celery actually suppresses and decreases stomach acid secretion.* Thus not much can be said about the statement: "the mineral salts found in celery juice increase the production of the undiscovered seven-acid blend of hydrochloric acid in the stomach". Bottom line, if you are deficient in stomach acid, celery will make you more so.

References

Alhowiriny, T. F et al. (2014). Gastric antiulcer, antisecretory and cytoprotective properties of celery (Apium graveolens) in rats. *Planta Medica, 80*(10). doi: 10.1055/s-0034-1382461

McMullen, M. K., Whitehouse, J. M., & Towell, A. (2015). Bitters: time for a new paradigm. *Evidence-based complementary and alternative medicine: eCAM, 2015,* 670504 doi:10.1155/2015/670504

Part 4

CONCLUSION

Final Thoughts

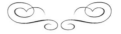

Celery is a member of one of the deadliest plant families on earth. A number of its close cousins, including hemlock and water hemlock, are lethal, while many others are to be strictly avoided. Celery is a medicinal herb that has been hybridized enough to change its chemical structure and take away its bitter, unpleasant taste. But we have outlined a range of very significant issues which might give one pause in over-doing—or even doing—celery.

Celery Integrated

We have food, and we have medicine. Variety and balance is the key in terms of eating. Unless there are allergies or sensitivities, celery may be a useful addition in normal amounts in salads, soups or a juicing regime, as a minor component with other ingredients. Juicing is hardly new, and its great advantage is the wide variety of different plant nutrients that can be garnered from beets, carrots, cucumber, lettuce, kale and scores of other vegetables and fruits. However, remember that the pesticide and heavy metal issue applies, and it is not clear that small doses are safe. Also, at a food dosage you will get just trace amounts of various bioactive ingredients—and that is a good thing. There is no need here to discuss the validity of various incomprehensible, miraculous claims. The whole of creation is a miracle. Celery is not more special than any other weed, fruit, tree or flying insect that partakes in this amazing life. Most of them, however, dont have 16 drawbacks.

Herbs vs Pharmaceuticals

It is clear. Celery is a herbal medicine that can be eaten occasionally as a food. It is not a nutritional supplement and in fact is very poor in body or health building nutrients. Its medicinal benefit lies in certain active ingredients. Some of those components, like apigenin, are a mixed bag, with toxicity to cells (cytotoxic) and liver (hepatotoxic), increased bleeding time, infertility effects, etc. Some are almost wholly toxic, like psoralens, but still have some drug application. In every instance of using a botanical medicine, there is a risk-benefit ratio, just as with medical drugs. The approach of the pharmaceutical and medical world is to find the active ingredients or therapeutic molecules and either extract them from a plant, or better yet, synthesize them. This is so that they can be made in adequate quantity, and for the dose to be precisely quantifiable. Plant content of active ingredient varies widely from plant to plant, place to place and season to season. The herbal world is an incredibly generous garden of healing possibilities. But we have to respect each plant for what it does and where it fits. Sometimes it is the whole, and sometimes the part that will benefit us the most. Even herbal companies try to find a balance between the whole and the part by assaying and "spiking" herbal products with their specific active ingredients.

Herbs in Context

In the early days of my practice, some 40 years ago, my naturopathic colleagues and I would (unkindly) jest about what was termed the "medical retreads" alluding to how one fixes up an old tire. Some mainstream doctors of the day had adopted a few natural therapeutics, such as herbs and nutritionals, but were looking at illness, disease and cure, in the same old way.

It was just another therapy, grafted onto a reductionist way of looking at the human body as a mechanical device, a car, just a machine, incapable of self-regulation, intelligent co-ordination and healing capacities. Without a holistic understanding of the healing process we are back in a round of superficial and symptomatic relief—even if using natural treatments. That is the backdrop of our current culture, as this superficial and expedient way of looking at health fits in with a world of easy fixes and advertising hype.

Plants, herbs, minerals and the natural substances they contain have the ability to improve and change our lives in a myriad of ways. In the right form and used in the right way, they can even move us towards listening both with our rational mind and our intuitive heart. That in turn can help brings us the wisdom to make sound choices. Those choices are like crossroads on our journey towards vibrant health.

It is my sincere wish that you may always choose wisely.

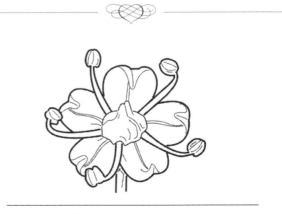

Typical Flower Form of Apiaceae

About the Author

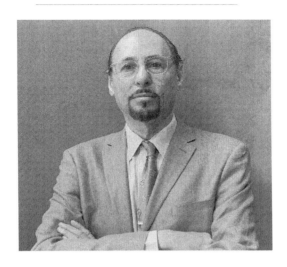

Dr Asa Hershoff ND has been practicing, writing and speaking about natural health and personal growth for 40 years. Pioneering Canada's natural health movement, he co-founded the Canadian College of Naturopathic Medicine in 1978. Since then he has traveled the globe rediscovering and connecting to healing truths scattered across time and culture. Asa integrates the wisdom of ancient healing traditions with modern science to help nurture the full spectrum of the human journey.

asahershoff.com
the5wisdoms.com
5elementenergyhealing.com
facebook.com/AsaHershoff/
youtube.com/c/AsaHersh

Scan me

INDEX

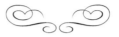

— A —

abdomen 33, 78

abortion 21, 60, 62

addicted 81

addiction 48

addictions 25

adrenal 48, 63, 85, 100

Aethusa 21, 23

alcohol 35, 47, 64

alkaloids 7, 10, 13, 19, 26

allergenic 32, 33, 35

allergy 9, 32-34, 36-37, 43-44, 62, 67, 75, 78

aluminum 72

Alzheimer's 57

anaphylaxis 32-34, 36, 43

anticancer 94

anti-microbial 99

antiviral 99

anxiety 25, 81

apigenin 60-61, 65-66, 69, 81, 90, 104-105, 111

apiole 69

Apiaceae 14-16, 22, 34, 38-39, 42, 44, 51, 53, 73, 82, 95-96, 101, 112 apoptosis 39

arsenic 27, 72-73

arteries 46, 50, 57

arthritic 16

artichokes 98, 103, 107

asparagus 88-89

aspirin 50, 65-66, 95

asthma 32-33, 36

— B —

B vitamins 88-89

bacteria 18, 27, 47, 55, 58

bergapten 39

bioactives 82, 94-95, 103-105, 110

bitters 107-108

bleeding Time 65, 111

blood sugar 63, 77, 100

brassica 49

breast 57, 89, 98

breastfeeding 61

broccoli 11, 98, 103

bruising 65

bullae 41, 43

burdock 106-107

— C —

cadmium 72-73

calcium 84, 88-89, 107

cancer 4, 8, 19, 21, 25, 27, 38, 42, 47, 48, 56-57, 59, 67, 74, 94, 96, 98, 102-105

carotenoid 87

carrot 11, 14, 18-19, 21, 32-34, 39, 87, 104, 110

cataract 42, 87

celeriac 17, 34, 40, 44

celery allergy 33-34, 36-37, 43-44, 67

chamomile 104

cheese 48, 89

cherries 13

chicken 40, 56, 89-90

cholagogue 106

cholesterol 25, 105

chromium 72

Cicuta 19-20, 51, 81, 93

cicutoxin 19

cinnamon 103, 107

Conium 19-20, 51, 81

cortisol 48

cucumber 110

curcumin (see turmeric) 9

cytochrome P450 46-49, 54

cytotoxic 8, 104, 111

— D —

dandelion 106-107

diarrhea 25, 63, 78, 105

digestion 16, 78, 107

diuretic 10, 16, 51, 63, 100-101

drug interactions 50

— E —

eczema 25

elderly 21, 64, 100, 107

element 15, 17, 52, 74, 80

embryo 60, 62

enzymes 46, 48-49, 84

estrogen 48, 61

exhaustion 63, 85

— F —

falcarinol 104

fennel 16, 39

ferritin 103

fetal abnormalities 4, 60

flavonoid 26, 98, 104

foodstuff 4, 8, 9, 55-57, 86, 103

fruits 6, 8-9, 13, 44, 70, 86, 105, 110

fungicide 39, 44

furanocoumarins 36, 39-41, 43-44, 104

— G —

garlic 88, 105

genotoxic 104

gentian 106-107

geriatric 87

ginger 106-107

ginkgo 72, 101

glucosides 7, 10, 26

goldenseal 106

grapefruit 50

— H —

headache 4, 42, 77, 100

heartburn 78

health claims 24

heavy metals 4, 22, 62, 72-74, 81, 90-92, 110

hemlock 19-22, 51, 93, 110

hemophilia 50, 65

henbane 7, 13, 15

heparin 50

herpes 42, 99

high blood pressure 101

hogweed 39-40, 45

homeopathy 27, 75, 114

H. pylori 18

hyoscyamus 95

— I —

immune system 34, 46, 72, 87, 90, 99, 102

Infants 57, 61

infarction 64

Infection 16, 63, 99

influenza 99

insomnia 4, 42, 77

insulin 100

ischemia 101

— J —

jaundice 16

juicing 34, 41, 77, 110

— K —

keratosis 42

kidneys 22, 63, 69, 72, 73, 87, 91

— L —

lactation 62

L-dopa 94

lead-zinc 74

lemons 98

lettuce 11, 87, 98, 110

leukemia 27, 57

light sensitivity 22, 38, 90

lithium 52

lutein 87, 92

luteolin 26, 98, 104

low Blood Pressure 51, 63

— M —

macular 87

magnesium 84, 89

male fertility 107

miscarriage 4, 22, 60

mastic gum 18

melanoma 42

melatonin 88

mental 27, 52, 81

mercury 72-73

mugwort 32, 44

— N —

nerves 41

nervous 8, 41, 50-51, 53

neurotoxic 19, 21, 81

niacin 5

nitrates, nitrites 35, 55-57, 59, 90

— O —

obesity 67-68

oranges 21, 86

oregano 98

ovaries 59, 79

— P —

pancreas 57, 100

pantothenic acid 84-85, 88

pyridoxine 88, 121

Parkinson's 94, 101

parsley 15, 18, 21-23, 33-34, 39, 49, 54, 69, 73

parsnips 14, 18, 34, 39

peppers 86, 98

pesticides 47, 70-71, 81, 90, 110

pharmaceuticals 48-51, 75, 111

pheromone 28

phosphorus 84

phototoxic 41, 43

phthalides 81, 102

phytophotosensitivity 21, 38, 41

pituitary 61, 68

platelet 65-66

potassium 55, 84, 89-91

potato 8, 13, 15, 87-88, 90

pregnancy 60-62

prostate 103

protein 8, 57, 90, 105, 107

psoralens 39-42, 44, 90, 99, 111

psoriasis 25, 40, 44

pyridoxine 88

— R —

reflux 18

retina 87

riboflavin 84, 88, 121

Rosaceae 13

rosemary 9

Rutaceae 39, 44

— S —

sacrum 79

salads 98, 110

salami, sausage 55, 56

scurvy 86

seafood 90

seaweed 89

sedative 11, 53

seizures 4, 19, 52, 95

serotonin 88

shiitake 89

sleepiness 53

smallage 15, 17

smoking 48, 55

sodium 55, 57, 64, 89, 91-92

spices 9, 12, 14, 22, 70

spinach 71, 73, 87-90

spirulina 90

spleen 16

squash 87

stomach 18, 57, 59, 65, 78, 103, 107-108

stroke 9, 50, 63-64, 66, 101-102

sunburn 38, 41

superfoods 9

suppression 46, 48, 61, 107

— T —

thyroid 2, 52, 59, 67-68

tobacco 13, 30, 57

tomato 13, 15, 35, 64, 89

toothache 15

truffles 28

tumors 102-103

turmeric (see curcumin) 9, 103, 106

— U —

ulcers 18

umbelliferae 14, 18, 37, 80 (see Apiaceae)

urinary 58, 63, 71, 78

urticaria 33, 78

— V —

vitamin C 2, 58, 84-86

vitamin E 58

vitamin K 84, 88

vitiligo 38, 40, 44

vomiting 10, 33, 41

— W-Z —

water dropwort 21-22, 51

willow 7, 95

wrinkles 38, 42

zeaxanthin 92

zinc 90

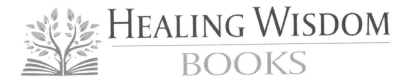
HEALING WISDOM
BOOKS

FORTHCOMING IN 2020

The Scar Cure

The first book to detail the remarkable ability of homeopathic, herbal and nutritional protocols to help remove, decrease and prevent scarring in any area of the body.

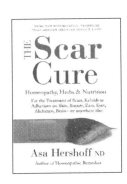

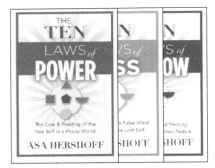

The Ten Laws

The books that explain the 3 phases of being that determine our happiness, our suffering, our being a lost soul, part of the dark side, or a fully empowered and connected individual.

..

https://www.healingwisdombooks.com
https://www.asahershoff.com

info@healingwisdombooks.com

321 N Pass Ave, Ste 151
Burbank, CA 91505

925-5WISDOM (925) 594-7366

SCAN ME

Books from Asa

Homeopathic Remedies

The definitive guide to the top 10 homeopathic treatments for 100 different conditions, with a concise and clear introduction to homeopathic principles, unique anatomical-remedy diagrams & accurate prescribing information.

Avery-Penguin 319 pp 2000

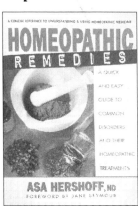

Herbal Remedies

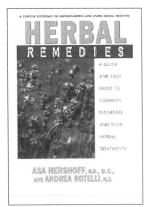

A concise, comprehensive guide to the top 10 or so herbs for 76 conditions, with anatomy-herb diagrams & principles of herbal medicine.

Avery-Penguin 343 pp 2001

Homeopathy for Musculoskeletal Healing

This is the only accurate guide to the homeopathic treatment and cure of injuries, joint, ligament and tendon problems throughout the body. With 61 remedies, the book covers headache, back pain, arthritis and more.

North Atlantic Books. 314 pp. 1996

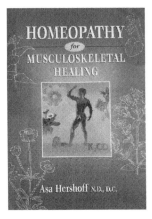

Manufactured by Amazon.ca
Bolton, ON